I … VE

A CE… OF BRITISH LINKS … H THE CHRISTIAN MEDICAL COLLEGE & HOSPITAL VELLORE, INDIA

Edited by

CLARE HOWES

Published by CCH. 2000

Printed by OCP, Old Oxted, Surrey RH8 9JJ

To Christopher, Cathy, Rob and Ben
whose lives have been intertwined with my involvement
in Vellore and whose support has been invaluable.

A Century of British Links with CMCH Vellore

CONTENTS **Page**

Foreword *Clare Howes* **1**

The 1920s

Miss Vera Pitman : CMCH 1928–1962
Eirene Mills & George Pitman **11**

The 1930s

Vellore Hospital in the 1930s : a patient's view
Gladys Bevan **14**

Married at Vellore 1937 : given away by Dr Ida
Gwendoline Skinner **16**

The 1940s

A Pharmacist's View 1946-1956 *Eirene Mills* **25**

Dr Robert Cochrane : Director 1944-1948 *Newsletter* **31**

The Right Revd Lesslie Newbigin *Clare Howes* **33**

James McGilvray CMCH 1942-1944 *Newsletter* **34**

A Short Memoir of my time at Vellore 1940s-1950s
Paul Brand **35**

Our Early Years at Vellore *Margaret Brand* **45**

The 1950s

Radiologist at Vellore 1951-1964 *Donald Paterson* **49**

A Dietician in Vellore 1940s-1950s *Helen Butler* **52**

Albert Jefcoate : Vellore Concerts 1951 onwards
Roger Jefcoate & Eric Gardner **55**

Page

Margaret Nash CMCH 1948-1965

Eirene Mills & Linnet Smith **58**

The Somervell Connection *Jim Somervell* **61**

CMCH 1953-1971 *John Webb* **63**

Memoirs of a Wife, Mother, School Founder and Doctor

Alison Webb **70**

Memoirs of CMCH Vellore *Robert Balfour* **77**

The 1960s

Happy Days at CMCH as a Dietician 1961-1969

Ruth Angove **81**

Engineering and Public Relations 1962-1983

Ann & Brian Witchalls **85**

Anaesthetist 1963-1967 *Margaret Riddoch* **89**

Reminiscences of a Physician 1962-1972 *Jim Milledge* **91**

Looking from the Outside 1964-1971 *Peter Bishop* **97**

Dr Valerie Major : Anaesthesiology 1967-1995

Clare Howes **103**

Memories of an Occupational Therapist 1966-1993

Monica Hopkins **103**

Memories of a Pharmacist 1967-1983

Rosemary Murchie **107**

Thirty years as part of the CMCH Family 1968-1998

Ann Bothamley **113**

OT at CMCH 1968-1983 *Jean Bald* **115**

		Page
The 1970s		
An Anaesthetist at Vellore 1969-1972	*Ruth Mansfield*	**117**
Dr Ruth Mansfield MBE	*Clare Howes*	**118**
The Vellore Concerts	*David Chesterman*	**120**
The Revd Joe Pratt : St John's 1974-1992	*Valerie Major*	**122**
The US Ambassador at Big Bungalow 1979	*Peter & Christine Hill*	**123**
The 1980s		
Lord Coggan and Lord Runcie	*Clare Howes*	**125**
Vellore Service : Radiation Physicist 1981-1983	*Christopher Green*	**126**
The 1990s		
Young Volunteers in the 1990s at CMCH	*Dominic Jenkin & David Keown*	**132**
Speech Therapist 1993-1994	*Amanda Howett*	**135**
Memories of an Archivist 1995	*Oliver Wooller*	**137**
British Personnel in the 21st Century :		
The Flemings	*Newsletter*	**139**
Other staff	*Clare Howes*	**140**

FOREWORD

"In my end is my beginning" T. S. Eliot - Four Quartets

The celebration of the centenary of the Christian Medical College and Hospital, Vellore is an appropriate time to look back at the links between Vellore in India and Britain and Ireland. I chose the word *"links"* in the title deliberately, because I see the contributions made by people from countries around the world as the links of a circular chain, which began at Vellore one hundred years ago. The success of CMCH at the end of its first century is directly linked to the strength of its founding spirit: over the years all the staff, including the British staff and volunteers, have been the links to that spirit of the past and to its future continuation. The testimonies of the British staff will show how the overseas links over the years all connect to the spirit of the beginning of CMCH. The effective end of overseas staff service of the kind described by the bulk of the contributors, is merely the beginning of another stage of CMCH's history, when overseas links are different but still valued.

The word *"links"* perhaps suggests too defined a connection; it would be better to describe the links between Britain and Vellore as *"tentacles"*. This better conveys the subtle spread of influence extending in both directions. For instance, when my late Mother was desperately ill some years ago and I had set up a Friends of Vellore office in the corner of her Hospital room, the Doctor who finally effected a cure had worked at CMCH years before. In my eighteenth year as Director of the Friends of Vellore, I have grown accustomed to the fact that almost everyone I meet will have some link, however distant, with Vellore.

Staff at CMCH and Friends of Vellore in Britain know of my interest in the archives and in the history of the institution and its supporting groups overseas. I began by organising the Archives of the British Friends of Vellore, which are now stored in the India Section of the British Library. We then commissioned from a senior British archivist a feasibility study of the task of preserving CMCH's Archives and we sent out a British archivist to undertake this. All went well until, on my first visit to the CMCH Archive, I found that there were no papers from the crucial 1900-1947 period! I instigated a search for these, without success, but I did find some early visitors' books and photographs in the Scudder Room that should now have been incorporated into the Archives at CMCH.

It was partly because of my regret at the gaps in the archive record, that I started to encourage the British staff to make a record of their time at CMCH and I suggested that the Friends of Vellore should present these records to CMCH Vellore as a tribute to mark its centenary.

I undertook this task with the deference due from an Oxford English graduate who was aware that the CMCH staff present and past could write far better than me. It was also salutary for me, as a former BBC Announcer, to discover when attending CMCH Councils, the fluency and eloquence of the staff when saying "*just a few words*". In the same way, having learnt my administrative skills while working for the Civil Service, I have been impressed by seeing busy medical staff coping so efficiently with the organization of CMCH.

It is important to recognize that what follows are the memoirs of British staff and others with close CMCH connections: in no way are they official histories, although important for recording the personnel and changes throughout the last century.

There are also gaps in the contributions; it has always been difficult to pin down Elective Students and Volunteers – some of whom do not come through official channels. It is also difficult to find information about earlier British staff, although the early CMCH records seem to show that British staff and visitors were there from the beginning of the Institution.

Despite much cajolement on my part over several years and having filled some gaps by extrapolating items from previous newsletters, some British staff could not be persuaded to put pen to paper. However, "*Full many a flower is born to blush unseen*," and we are appreciative of the unrecorded service they gave.

Friends of Vellore office staff have also served CMCH from Britain. It is to be regretted that my predecessor was not able to contribute an account of the Friends of Vellore office over the three decades she was in post. The Friends of Vellore organisation in Britain, as I outlined to CMCH Staff at Council a few years ago, began in the 1940s and there have been many dedicated staff, such as Majorie Pearson, working for the Office. I can only speak of the last two decades while I have been Director of the Friends of Vellore and when both Muriel Skey and Sue Lowndes worked in the Office for over 10 years and Sue Chipchase has valiantly rendered these accounts legible.

It is also important to record the contributions of all the British Friends of Vellore over the years who have their own links with CMCH; some, like our Hon. Treasurer, have served for many years on F.O.V. Committees. They have enabled the Fellowship between Britain and Vellore to continue growing. The Christian Medical College and Hospital, Vellore and its staff have been featured in many books written and published in Britain and I have added these to our Archives in the British Library.

The links, or tentacles, of Vellore continue to increase: a few years ago a distant British cousin of Dr Ida Scudder visited CMCH, aged 82, as part of a Pilgrimage group; a donation was sent from a father whose son received help from CMCH, 25 years ago after a road accident. My elder son ran the Friends of Vellore office when I was last at Vellore and my younger son worked in Rehabilitation as a volunteer. Young medical students and volunteers continue to approach me and so the stories will continue. As the Isleta Indians say: "*when the stories are no longer told, there will no longer be a need for them*".

The freshness and humour of the memoirs which follow, demonstrate the reciprocal respect and affection between Britain and CMCH Vellore. As Kevin Lynch wrote: "*A sense of the stream of time is more valuable and poignant and engaging than a formal sense of remote periods*".

The British Friends of Vellore offer these memoirs, to mark the Centenary of that great Institution The Christian Medical College and Hospital, Vellore.

Clare Howes
London
May 2000

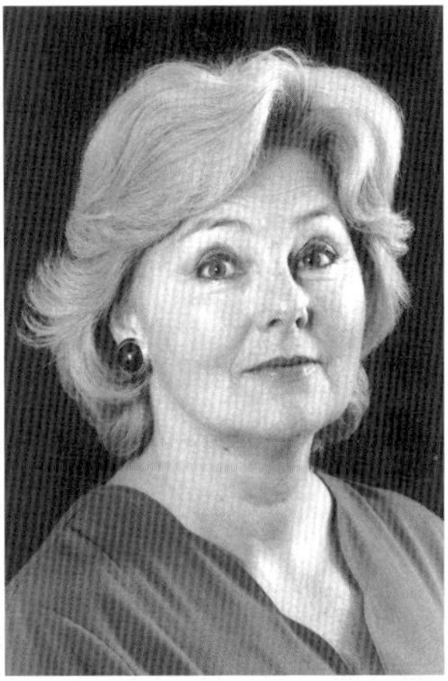

The 1920s

Miss Vera Pitman. CMCH 1928-1962

Vera Pitman was Nursing Superintendent at CMCH from 1928 to 1962. Sadly she died only a few months after she retired to the UK following 34 years' service at Vellore and the following memories are from:

1. *CMCH Council Minutes,*
2. *Mrs Eirene Mills and*
3. *Her nephew Mr George Pitman*

1. "Miss Vera Pitman graduated in General Nursing and Midwifery from Guy's Hospital, London, in 1925. She came to Vellore by chance as she was originally assigned to missionary service in China. We thank God for so graciously directing her here, for it was surely his Divine purpose for this institution to have guided her to Vellore. The School of Nursing could not have produced the graduates it did without her wise guidance, local support and encouragement. She held nearly every office both in Nursing Service and the School of Nursing.

Her interest was not in the organization as such but in how these State and National organizations can contribute to the development of the nurse as an individual. She revised the Handbooks of the T.N.A.I. in 1958 and assisted with and edited other text books like the New Text Book for Nurses in India, volumes I and II.

Thus she was compelled to live a busy life but never lacked time to speak to a discouraged nurse, filling her with hope and courage, and to pay a visit to her students when they were sick at the hospital. Her true greatness and largeness of heart can be seen in the way she methodically educated others to replace her out of every office she held. She produced disciples to hold even greater responsibilities than she had.

We record with gratitude our appreciation of her unostentatious but most significant contribution to Vellore."

CMCH Council Minute 1962

2. "Miss Vera Pitman was a woman of rare qualities. She had the grace to retire from her position as Nursing Superintendent when she felt it right for an Indian colleague to take her place. Further, she had the strength of character not to interfere in any way but supported her successor as a loyal colleague and helped her to shoulder the responsibility in her own way. She was always interested in young people. As the Nurses said, in their farewell address to her, she had the willingness to consider suggestions from junior staff and students in spite of her long experience. She was not only a womanof ability but also had the important gift of leadership. She had enthusiasm and an infectious gaiety, which kept her young in mind and spirit. When I first went out as a very raw recruit, she never tried to impose her ideas on me but while always ready to help, left me to make my own decisions and judgments.

When she invited me to live with her in her tiny house, I became even more aware of her rare humility and her great sense of humour which made light of her handicap of deafness and any other difficulty.

Young and old respected her, loved her and confided in her. She had high ideals and was determined that she should not have more comforts than others just because she had held a high position. Because of a true graciousness of spirit she never made others feel ill at ease even though they were somewhat keener on the material things of life. Only those who knew her well realized just how she lived. In fact, she was a rare woman and it is impossible to do justice to her qualities in a short appreciation.

Her life of dedication has been like a torch lighting the way of nurses, students, colleagues and young missionaries, and although now her torch is out, yet others whom she helped and influenced will be carrying on the light which she gave to them."

Eirene Mills

3. Vera Pitman was my aunt. I have lived with Vellore from earliest times, whether it was her rare furloughs, bringing wooden elephants or the Indian nurses who passed through my grandparents' and parents' homes.

It was a great thrill for me to visit Vellore briefly and to see Pitman Road and more especially to meet very senior ladies who had been taught by her.

George Pitman

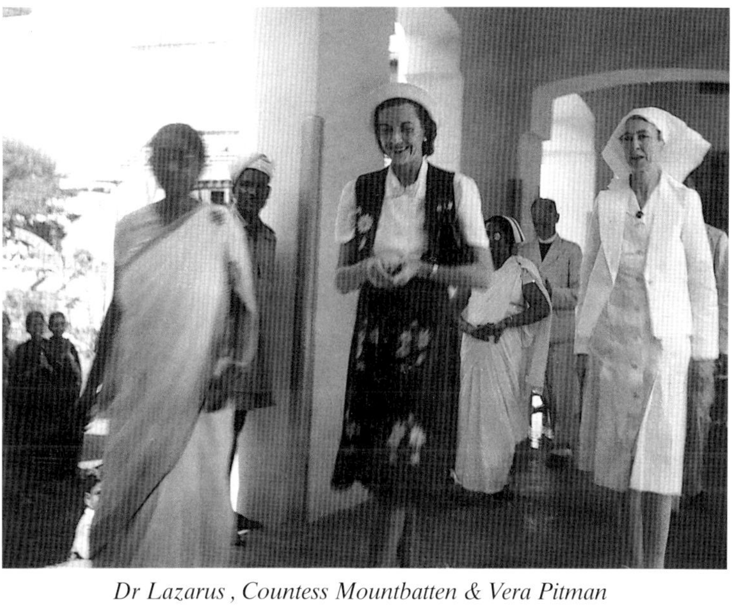

Dr Lazarus , Countess Mountbatten & Vera Pitman

The 1930s

Vellore Hospital in the 1930s: A Patient's View

by Mrs G Bevan

I began my missionary service in Medak, Nizam's Dominions, now Andhra Pradesh, and lived in the ladies' bungalow in a large compound with six other women missionaries. I was in charge of the Girls' Training School.

When I became ill, it was decided that I should go to Vellore in South India, which was the place we turned to when special medical aid was necessary. A colleague was asked to accompany me and she also benefited from the experience.

How can one describe our amazement when we came to a great white building set in the typical unhygenic village street of those days? I marvel as I see it all now, the vision of one dedicated person, Dr Ida Scudder, who conceived and brought into being this vast centre of healing.

We were taken upstairs to a white ward, shining in its welcome. I lay in bed, grateful to be there, and then in came Dr Ida herself with her colleague. She was short in stature in comparison to the other taller and younger doctor. Their decision was that I was too ill for them to give me the help I needed and that I should return home to England! Plans were made and this was the end of my contact with Vellore for some time.

During a year or so at home I spent time in two London hospitals and was put down as a neurotic. At the second, a younger doctor came with the older one who was attending me and said quietly, "*I think I could have helped you if I had been there*". That encouragement meant a great deal.

A friend in India (I guessed who), sent money for me to have a holiday which was renewing and encouraging. After a while I said to my mother, "*I think I can go back*".

Again in Medak in charge of the Girls' Boarding School, living in the same bungalow I found myself again needing help. Vellore! I asked to see a doctor I had heard did wonders for people suffering from all kinds of diseases. After diagnosing amoebic dysentery, she put me on a diet and would come in and say, "*Have you drunk all that*?" pointing to a kooja on the window sill – this was a delightfully shaped vessel which everyone used for water. This diet is still mine today in my 90s at the end of the century!

Some time later, I married and was expecting a little one when once again we turned to Vellore. I was asked to make the three day journey in January 1939. Ann was expected in March but because of my medical history they wished to keep a check on me and suggested I stay until she came. I sat for weeks on the flat roof of the hospital in the sunshine, sewing the little garments, enjoying the peace, care and assurance this gave me. I could look down on the beautiful roof of the Chapel which was the inspiration of all Vellore's ministry.

I knew Sister Vera Pitman on the staff and was told she had gone away for the day just as Ann was telling us she was coming! Suddenly, Sister Vera came in wearing her outdoor clothes – she had asked about me on her return and came at once when she heard the news. This shows the concern the staff felt for their patients at Vellore. She went away and changed and there she was in the theatre holding my hand – I nearly crushed hers she told me afterwards!

All went well and the time was nearing our home-going when I noticed Ann had changed colour. In a few minutes, the specialist was with us but fortunately all was well. This is another instance of the wonderful care given to the patients at Vellore.

Later on, we were staying in Medak in the vast bungalow with staff to supervise and guests to entertain on special occasions. I also had full care of Ann, who was about two years old, when, one day, I began to tremble from head to foot. A friend in another place kindly took Ann into her home with her little boy and her older sister – where we knew she would be cared for. I went to Vellore – where else? But they told me they could do nothing for me. I told them of a doctor further south in the Swedish Hospital who helped people in wonderful ways. "*May I go there?*" "*Go and come back to tell us*", they said at Vellore. I went and was completely healed. The doctor who helped me became a good friend and later came to see us in Somerset whenever she came to our country. I went back to Vellore and told them what had happened – I trust someone else benefited from my experience.

These are pictures of Vellore in the past, but we know that many people are receiving the same kindness and healing today.

Married At Vellore 1937: "Given Away" by Dr Ida

by the late Gwendoline Skinner (née Sands)

We sailed from Liverpool on 20th September 1935 on the City of Cairo. The voyage took three weeks, and we were destined for Cochin. After a meal with friends, we took the train to Katpadi Station, where we duly arrived at four o'clock in the morning. Miss Pitman and another nurse met us. I was taken to the Hospital, but for Martyn it was the Medical College for the night, or what remained of it.

Next day I was immediately into uniform and met the other people living in the bungalow, doctors and nursing sisters, and went to the maternity wards where I would be working. My bedroom was, in fact, next to the Labour Rooms.

The missionary and medical staff at Vellore were mixed national and denominational people. There were four of us nurses and we lived at the Hospital. Miss Dell Haughton was the Senior Sister. She was an elderly American who looked after the housekeeping in the Bungalow, was in charge of the servants, did some admin-istrative work, and looked after linen etc. in the hospital. Miss Vera Pitman was, of course English, Guys, and a Methodist. Miss Lorna Chute, a Canadian from Toronto, and Baptist. And then me, English, Guys and L.M.S.

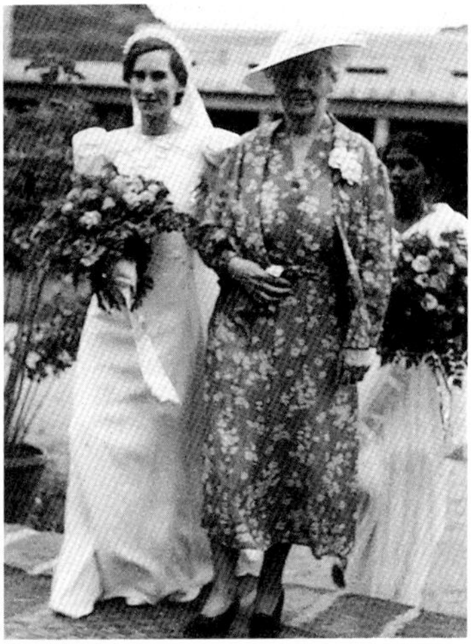

Miss Sands arriving with Dr Ida

Vera lived in the Nurses' Home and was largely responsible for their wellbeing. She was in charge of the large medical ward, most of the teaching of the nurses and also of engaging new nursing recruits year by year. Lorina lived in the Bungalow and was Theatre Sister in charge of Surgical and Gynae. Wards. I think she and Vera looked after the Children's Wards, taught practical midwifery, delivered babies and tutored the 'midder' class, preparing them for the British Midwifery exam. I also taught infant care and feeding, and the care of premature babies, which I specialised in.

There were two staff nurses, one in each of the wards. Downstairs was the so-called 'septic ward' where patients were admitted, who had not attended the ante-natal clinics at the hospital. These patients often had been terribly mishandled by the old 'barber women' in their homes, and were often badly infected. Upstairs was the nice 'clean' ward with patients admitted in labour after antenatal care.

There seemed a large contingent of doctors. First and foremost was Doctor Ida Scudder, whose great dream-come-true was this hospital. She lived with her friend and benefactor Miss Gertrude Dodd in their spacious bungalow at College Hill. Then her niece, Doctor Ida B Scudder, lived at the hospital and was in charge of the obstetrics with me and also ran the X-Ray Department. Doctor Ida was nearing her 70th year but still very active in operating on women, mostly European but also wealthy Indians from all over India. She specialised in Gynaecology. Next was Dr Finlay Jessie, a Canadian surgeon who lived at the Medical

College. Dr Jefferson, also a Canadian, was largely teaching the medical students and her friend was Dr Graham, a physician from Scotland, who largely cared for the Children's Ward. They lived in the hospital Bungalow, as too did Dr Innis the Senior Physician who hailed from Australia (a bossy woman!). Two new doctors joined after me, Dr Bernie Seibers and Dr Ena Brown, and started off in the Bungalow later moving to College Hill. A charming young doctor from South Carolina came as temporary staff and she and I were great friends. She was Gladys Morgan (after leaving she married a Scot and we met her in Kotagiri with her baby William and mine, Alyson).

Oh, and then there was Dr Jeffery who specialized in Eyes. Unfortunately she had been in a sanatorium with T.B. and was about to live permanently in the hills at Kotagiri. There were several medical doctors, Vellore trained, on the staff. One, Dr Ebline Thomas, was in my department and we came to blows re student nurses delivering babies, unheard of in the USA and the reason I, as a British nurse, was there. Her husband was the Hospital Chief Administrator and came to my aid regarding problems of all sorts, re money and other personal things, a very delightful person. Nurse Petrie was in charge of the Pharmacy and in charge of the Pharmacological students. She was a Scottish Presbyterian and lived in the Bungalow.

The hospital rooms were spread over a large area and were mainly two storied buildings. The entrance was through large gates into a big forecourt and then there was an attractive portico with antigium and bourganvilia over it, leading to the front hall. Above the entrance was a small clock tower. The Maternity Wing was to the left and behind and to the right, was Out-Patients and then the Medical Ward above. Private rooms were facing the front on the first floor between Clean Maternity and Medical and along the outer corridor, near the Children's Ward. There were raised covered pavements separating wards and departments, so the layout was quite spacious; the little Chapel was in the central court. An avenue of sweet scented cork trees led to our Bungalow and the Nurses Home to the right of it and lovely golden mahr trees surrounded these buildings.

Every morning there were prayers in the Chapel before going on duty. The nurses sat on rush mats on the tiled floor and staff sat on the raised pavement round them. A staff member conducted the little service, taking turns week-by-week, and Martyn often helped me when it was my turn, although I did feel I could manage after Carey Hall. I also had to take a Bible Class with the night nurses, in their special screened quarters, away over the roof from the main wards. All wards were modern and open with airy verandas and the 'talties' sun blinds to lower for sun and rain.

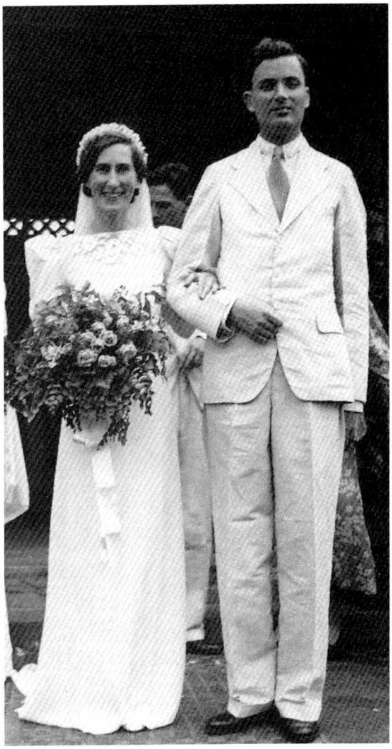

Mr & Mrs Skinner

The Labour Ward was, of course, my special domain and I would be there to instruct the students. When an urgent case came in the night, I was called and also the student who was getting her required number of cases. When there was a caesarean in the Main Theatre, I would be there to care for the baby and resuscitate it (often this was necessary for I found many blue babies!) I saw some horrific things with patients who came in after fearful mishandling outside and terrible septic cases; one girl with gangrene of the pelvis.

Then again, there was 'fun and games' in the wards when relations came and camped under the beds and Muslim women hid beneath their sheets and always demanded corner beds with screens. Relatives often fed the patient and there were facilities for them to cook in the compound: even so, I caught one family about to light a fire under the bed! Baby feeding was also quite a problem and the old grandmothers would smuggle in awful, dirty, little tin teapots and attempt to feed the baby.

There were our 'hospital babies' too. These were unwanted children, mostly girls, like Susheela, whose mother died from heart failure when she was born and others brought to us when rescued from, for example, being thrown into the village well. We cared for them in the maternity private rooms and tried to have them adopted. Sukinitala was a great favourite, very dark skinned and certainly an 'outcaste' child, but so sweet natured. (A Christian family had her.) Vinnala was fair skinned and a Muslim child. Varantha was rescued as illegitimate. We were able to find them homes.

Miriam and I 'adopted' Susheela, her father had five daughters and left her to us. He was a 'caste sudra' farmer. We had her baptized in our Chapel by the Indian Pastor of St John's Church. She was Susheela Grace Kantha Swami. At two years old she went to a nursery in Kolar, run by an American woman and then on to kindergarten and school and eventually married Samuel Moses, a good Methodist man with a good job in Bangalore. They have three children, two girls and a boy and keep in touch. Miriam adopted Susie outright when I left India.

Twice a week, a hospital 'bus', a kind of ambulance, went out on the roadside, stopping at known places where patients met them to receive regular injections to cure or retard their leprosy. Other ill people with minor complaints were treated and accident victims might be taken on to go to hospital. A doctor, nurse and pharmacist went with these 'buses'. Their destination on the routes were small clinics manned by an Indian doctor from the hospital. I accompanied the 'bus' on two occasions.

During my two years at Vellore, I had several weekend leaves and was able to visit Madras and Bangalore and met Martyn there. Our LMS and other friends were most kind, inviting us to stay during our engagement period, especially Revd and Mrs George Parker; he was Secretary for the Field in India and she was a sweet motherly soul. They met my parents in England on furlough when in Maidenhead later on.

I also visited Martyn in Gooty. I met L J Thomas (with whom

Martyn lived for his first year), Miss Mabel Few, Jack and Helen Rolles and Shirley, Freddie and Ethel (John she likes to be called) Malthus-Smith, Elizabeth and six months old Stephen. We climbed the Gooty Rock. This is an ancient fortification very nice, with lookouts over the countryside. There is a similar fortified hill just by the hospital at Vellore, which has French fortifications and the Vellore Fort, an enclosed fort in which are a Christian church, Muslim mosque and a Hindu temple, not in use then as it was desecrated, so one could go into the sacred inner court. In the fort was the Police Officers' Training College and Mr Horace Furness was in charge. There were lovely horses and we nurses and doctors were invited to ride them in some off-duty time. A most enjoyable pursuit! The Furnesses were English and became firm friends, especially as Eveline came to have her baby girl in my maternity department and she so kindly laid on my wedding reception at College Hill later on.

I had two holidays in the Hills in the hot weather in May whilst at Vellore. The first at Kotagiri, where Martyn also stayed in a boarding house. The second was in Kodaikanal, where we were able to stay in the High Clerc School. During these holidays we met and got to know many missionaries from all over South India especially Americans in Kodai, where the school is American. Many L.M.S. children went there too, including the Scopes, Firths, Cuttings and Wightmans. In Kodai, we enjoyed lovely walks through the woods to Pillar Rocks and climbing Perival to watch the sunrise. From Cokers Walk you look down to the Plains far below. There was the Anglican Church and the American United Church, where Martyn played the organ. An organisation called the Community Chest arranged concerts, plays and a Gilbert and Sullivan operetta during the six week holiday period, also a large Exhibition and Sale of High Clerc school. All most sociable!

At Vellore, we staff members were invited to special celebrations such as the American 'Thanksgiving' by some Arcot Mission folk. I remember one dinner party with the table laid in the garden and fairy lights around. We ate roast turkey and then the inevitable pumpkin pie. A small hospital at Ranipet was run by Dr Scudder's brother and was the original Scudder family parents' hospital where Ida started from. He was Dr Galen Scudder, after the great physician Claudius Galen!

My two years were nearing the end and our wedding date was fixed for 13th November 1937. We were to be married in the Medical College Chapel at Vellore, and our L.M.S., Revd George Parker had agreed to marry us, while Dr Ida would give me away, which she was very excited about. I had asked my two Indian staff nurses to be our bridesmaids, Miriam Solomon and Kanthi Swamidas. Martyn asked Harry Wrightman, his Cambridge student friend, to be his best man. In the event, he could not do so, because his first baby, Eleanor, decided to arrive on that very day. Jack Rolles filled the gap very graciously. Crates of wedding presents had been arriving from England and the kind Parkers, back from furlough, brought my wedding cake which Auntie Lizzie had made for me.

My family sent some beautiful ivory brocade material, ivory lace and a Vogue pattern for my dress. I had it made by a French dressmaker in Madras. A very lovely darned net veil was made by the Methodist Mission Lace Industry in Mysore. Bouquets for bride and bridesmaids were to come from Bangalore. We would spend our two week honeymoon on a tea and coffee plantation at Yercourt, a little hill station 3,000 feet up near Salem and would stay our first night with May Wilson there in Salem. Martyn and I chose our very fine rosewood furniture at the Arcot Mission Carpentry School nearby, at Katpadi. Vellore staff also gave us gifts of this furniture. We had purchased the two wedding rings in Madras the last time we met there. An eight-sided platinum one for me and a gold signet ring for Martyn.

I finished working a few days before the 13th, and was able to pack up my belongings, books etc. These, and two fine rush lounge chairs and an Indian carpet, would go to Kamala-puram right away. Our home would be the '*ladies*' (so-called) bungalow, where Martyn had '*camped*' this second year.

Martyn arrived at Vellore two days before the Revd and Mrs Parker, who arrived a day ahead of the wedding. He stayed at the

College and a 'rehearsal' was held. Dr Ida got me to go and spend an afternoon at her house to choose the dress she would wear at the ceremony, and I rested on her bed with her. She was so kind and thoughtful.

So my wedding day dawned and all was bustle and activity. When dressed in my bridal attire, I had to go and show it off to some of the private patients, nurses and so on. Some of them were coming by bus to the ceremony. Miss Dodd sent her large car for me and it was beautifully decorated inside and out with flowers: lovely tasselled hibiscus, roses etc. My bridesmaids were with me. The lovely College Chapel, beside the beautiful circular lotus pool, was decorated with pink and white flowers, with antigium and other climbers round the pillars. Martyn was there: so we were married and signed the L.M.S. register, which George Parker had brought.

As we left, masses of pink rose petals were showered on us by my nurses. Then there was the reception in the big College Hall with little tables for guests and a large table, up on a high dias for the wedding party. It was all a wonderful day. So, back to my room to change and then to Katpadi Railway Station with a great send off from friends and staff again. I wore a pretty green, brown and beige silk dress and brown straw hat, worn at my farewell service in London and kept for the occasion.

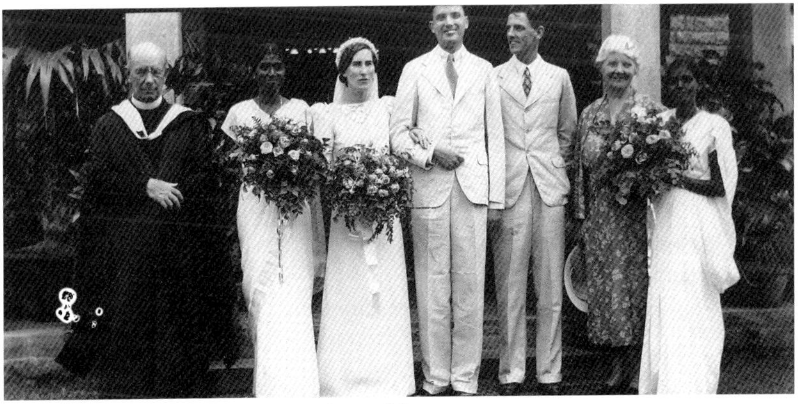

The wedding party

Farewell from Vellore Hospital 1937 to Gwendoline Sands on her marriage

Our Loving Sister Sands,

First of all we give our hearty thanks to you for coming to this hospital and helping us with your kind and good works.

We know that you have always undergone a lot of troubles to bring forth the high standard of nursing as well as midwifery. You have been discouraged so many times seeing the careless work of nurses and so many times we made you lose your temper. But we girls are very glad to see that sweet smile one or two minutes after that temper. We consider it as moon rising from darkness. Really it shows the purity of your mind and also your noble character.

We will never forget your presence during the morning rounds. You helped us to escape Doctor's scoldings, as you used to take the whole responsibility and so we were getting a narrow escape.

We are now very much afraid to tell our babies that their sweet mother is going to leave them, because we are sure that they will lose weight and have frequent motions.

Dearest sister, words fail to express our feelings of sorrow for your departure. But we are glad that you are going to enjoy a new life. We shall never forget you and your great help. Always we will remember you in our prayers. Let God shower his blessings on you

Your loving Nurses

NOTE

Mrs Skinner died this year and her children read part of the Nurses' letter, and Mrs Skinner's memoirs, at her funeral. They also asked for donations instead of flowers, which they sent to the Friends of Vellore. I hope they will derive some comfort from the thought that her memory will live on through the sharing of these memoirs.

CH

The 1940s

A Pharmacist's View 1946-1956

by Mrs Eirene Mills (née James)

I have been asked to write of my experiences at the Christian Medical College and Hospital, Vellore in order to indicate some of the many changes which took place from 1946 to 1956.

After graduating as B.Pharm (London) from Nottingham University during the war in 1942 and qualifying as a Pharmaceutical Chemist, I worked as an analytical chemist in British Drug Houses in London: I graduated as B.Sc (Chemistry) becoming a Fellow of the Pharmaceutical Society. This was followed by research on Vitamin C in Rose Hips at the Ovaltine Research Laboratories.

In 1945 I offered to join the Methodist Missionary Society but I was unsure whether my qualifications were needed on the Mission field. However, I was sent to Vellore as Chief Pharmacist and Lecturer to the medical students. It was such an exciting time to be working at CMC which had only recently been upgraded.

Dr Cochrane was the Director and the Revd James McGilvray the General Superintendent. In 1947 the first ten men Medical Students were admitted. 'M' Ward for private patients was started; before that there were a few private rooms opposite the corridor, which led to the X-Ray Department.

New staff kept arriving including Dr Paul Brand, the Orthopaedic Surgeon, the late Dr Reeve Betts, the first Chest Surgeon in India followed by Dr Jacob Chandy, the first Neuro Surgeon in India. At first there was one main operating theatre and a gynaecological theatre but when Dr Betts arrived, a new air-conditioned theatre was built followed by a further one for Dr Chandy. New Wards were also built for their patients; a blood bank had to be started for Dr Betts as he required 20 pints before he could do Lung Surgery. This was difficult at the start but the hospital was able to obtain blood from the political prisoners at the Jail in Vellore. Later when that supply failed, the Rickshaw men willingly contributed blood for a small fee, a cup of coffee and a piece of bread.

It was very exciting when Dr Paul Brand did his first operation to straighten the fingers of a Leprosy patient's hand. Also, but later, Dr R Howard Somervell, of Everest fame, came to work for a short time as Gastric Surgeon after retiring from Neyoor.

At first we sterilised pint bottles of IV Saline and IV Glucose Saline in the Pharmacy, which was then in one room, using a small autoclave heated by a Primus stove; later we were given a small room adjacent to the large pharmacy, which became my office and sterilizing room.

Over the years we had larger autoclaves and eventually an electric autoclave. All the rubber tubing, needles and bottles were cleaned in the Pharmacy by one of the Ward Aids, as we could not afford new tubing or bottles.

From time to time I had to make special injections for the ENT Department; the saline was tested for sterility and foreign particles on two rabbits which were kept in the Path Department; I had to inject the saline into their ears and take their temperatures.

Before the introduction of Dapsone for Leprosy patients, we sterilized Hydnocarpus oil in an electric oven for injection. This was taken out in the Roadside bus. Gold injections were still used for rheumatoid arthritis. There were about 12-14 Compounders (Dispensers) plus three Ward Aids and three Attenders; after a year I was joined by Miss Joyce Saunders MPS, who had previously worked at CMC.

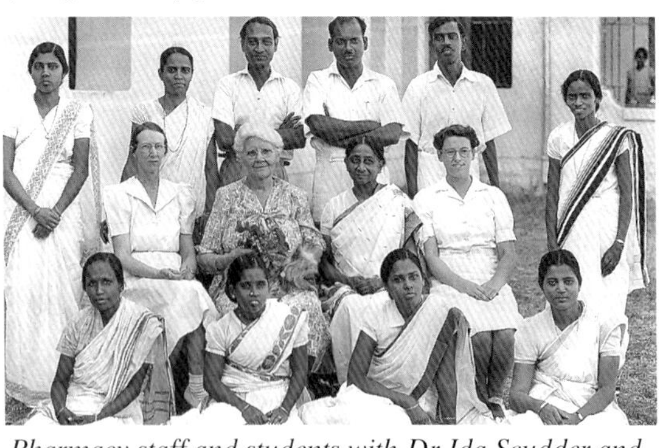

Pharmacy staff and students with Dr Ida Scudder and Dr H Lazarus

One compounder made up large Winchester Bottles full of various medicines; these could then be used immediately to dispense medicines to the Wards and Out-patients. When I first arrived, all the outpatients crowded around one large window; because there was no order, we had part of the Out-patient's courtyard enclosed, making two openings, one for women and one for men. Before we introduced this arrangement, the women had to wait until all the men had received their medicine! One dispenser worked full time on making the IV solutions and sterilizing them. We also had a storeroom outside and a full time store keeper.

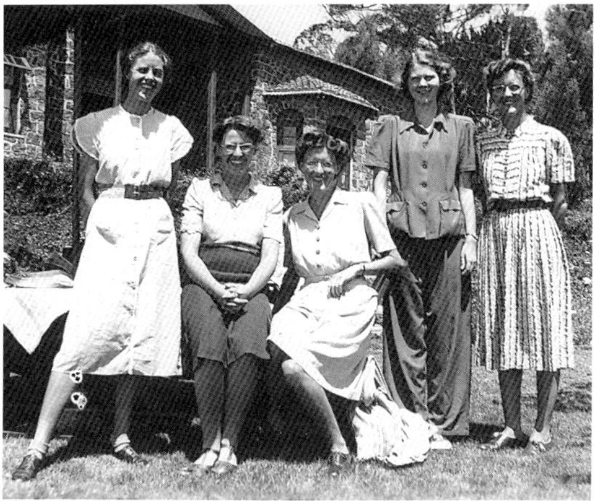

Miss Hutchinson, Miss James, Dr G Lewis and Miss M Simpson - 194?

Sometimes it was very difficult to obtain essential drugs, especially Penicillin and other injections. The Penicillin arrived in powder form in very small bottles; each day we had to add sterile water to 20 or 30 bottles which were then kept in a refrigerator ready for use. When empty, we used the bottles to make concentrated Glucose Saline to sell to other Mission Hospitals.

We had very little money to buy bottles for dispensing medicine, so the patients normally brought an assortment of containers, which was not very satisfactory. We did have Poison bottles, as I refused to dispense external lotions in any other containers. Our budget for drugs was less that a Lakh of Rupees and there was no cost accounting system.

The compounders used to be able to estimate by the look and clothes of a patient how much they were able to pay! However, with the help of the Revd James McGilvray, we obtained a large amount of Army Surplus Supplies from Avadi Military Stores.

The Doctors in Outpatients normally only prescribed four days' medicine as a precaution. We had labels printed in Tamil, Telegu and English but the compounders usually had to describe the amount by making an oval on the palm of their hands. In 1948 we produced a Hospital Pharmacopoeia for the use of the medical staff. We made our own pills and ointments, the latter often being dispensed on a small banana leaf or greaseproof paper, there were no tubes of ointment!

We did not make tablets but powders were dispensed by the conpounders weighing an exact amount and dividing it by a knife into the correct number of portions. We also made our own Plaster of Paris bandages in a small upstairs room. A Ward Aid worked full time rubbing the Plaster of Paris into gauze bandages.

Mr Joseph, one of the compounders, prepared the medicines for the Roadside Bus and went out with the doctor 3 times a week in a 30-mile radius. Each morning after prayers in the department, the Ward boxes were filled. We had to cover Night Calls and on Saturday and Sundays the dispensary was only open in the mornings but there was always a compounder on call.

We started a nursery school for the children of the Attenders and Ward Aids. Every morning a very small boy would collect milk from us, prepared from powdered milk sent from the USA. Besides teaching the Medical Students at the College twice a week, we trained about 10 Dispensing Students each year and taught the Nurses percentages etc.

When I first arrived in 1946 I lived in Ward C with three junior doctors; it was not very satisfactory and from time to time there were rats. Later I moved to the College but that was not suitable for working in the Hospital; eventually I was given a room in the Nurses' Hostel.

After furlough, I shared one of the four small houses behind the duplex with Vera Pitman. We had a small room each, a bathroom and a toilet at the end of the garden, which backed onto the wall of a house in the town.

Over the years it was a great joy to take part in the selection of Medical Students, as a Group Leader in charge of one of the tests. This was most interesting and rewarding. These tests were introduced by Dr Frank Lake who also prepared a pathology Museum filled with specimens. During this period, Dr Alexander Fleming, who first used Penicillin, visited the Hospital and gave a most interesting talk.

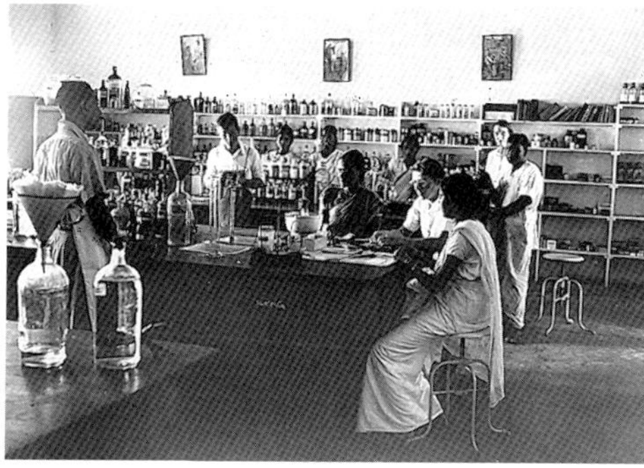
Hospital Dispensary

On the retirement of Dr Cochrane, Dr H Lazarus, who had worked as a Gynaecologist and Obstetrician for the government, became the Medical Superintendent and then Director. She was followed by Dr Carmen. Vera Pitman, the Nursing Superintendent, decided to resign and take a position in the College of Nursing so that Miss Anna Jacob could become Nursing Superintendent. After the Revd James McGilvray retired, the Revd H Shepherd, followed by General Wilson-Haffenden, were General Superintendents. Finally the Revd S Savarirayan took office.

A Men's Hostel was built on the College Campus and Dr E Gault became the first Dean of the men Medical Students. The men dispensing students lived in a house in Vellore town while the women students and unmarried women compounders lived in the Nurses' Hostel.

In 1947 India became Independent and there were great celebrations at the College and Hospital when the Indian flag was raised and the Indian National Anthem sung. This was later followed by a week of mourning when Mahatma Ghandi was assassinated. There was scarcely any violence in the town of Vellore when partition was announced; a few shops belonging to Muslims were boarded up for a day or two.

Also in September 1947, the Church of South India was inaugurated when Anglicans, Methodists, Congregationalists and Presbyterian's joined together to become a United Church. I was thrilled to be able to attend the service in Madras Cathedral. The two Tamil Speaking Churches, one S.I.U.C. and one S.P.G. and the English speaking Anglican Church St Johns (where the staff and students attended) all became part of the Church of South India. The full time

Chaplain of C.M.C., the Revd Dr A E Inbanathan was also a Minister of the C.S.I. and was Minister of St Johns for a period.

The overseas staff came from many countries during that period – America, Canada, Australian, England, Scotland, Wales, Ireland and Norway. Many different denominations and Missionary Societies were represented – C.M.S., S.P.G. (Anglican), Methodist, Presbyterian, Congregational, American Arcot Mission, Seventh Day Adventists, Orthodox Syrian Christian Church, Marthomite Church. CMCH was, and is, truly international and ecumenical.

In the winter months, Dr Ida Scudder would come down from Kodaikanal and do Ward rounds, followed by her little dog. She took part in all the celebrations for Independence Day.

There was a small Indian Pharmaceutical Society to which I belonged and I contributed a few items to their journal. Because of the regard Madras University had for CMCH over the years, I was involved in examining their students for a degree in Pharmacy.

It was a great privilege to work at CMCH and to have so many wonderful colleagues and be there at such an interesting time when the Hospital was expanding at a rapid rate and so many changes were taking place in India and in the Church. One of the highlights was the visit of Lady Mountbatten to the Pharmacy and another was when Pandit Nehru received lemonade at the gates of CMCH as he drove through the town after Independence.

In 1956 I had to return home unexpectedly for family reasons but CMCH and India will always have a special place in my heart.

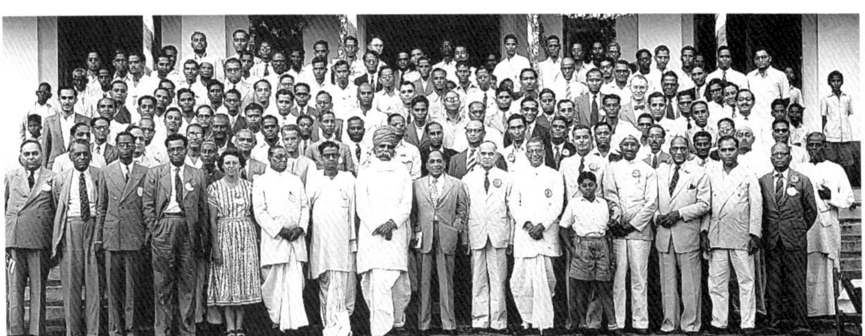

Indian Pharmaceutical Conference 1953: Miss James (5th on left front)

Dr Robert Cochrane

Principal of Vellore Medical School. Director CMCH 1944 - 1948

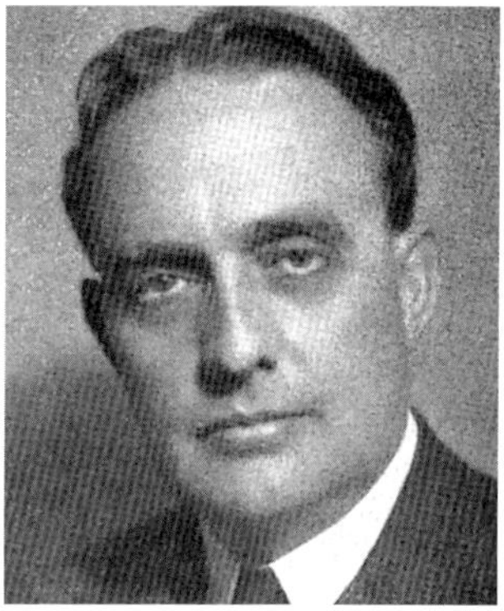

Dr Robert Cochrane

Dr Robert Cochrane, one of the world's leading Leprologists, died in August 1985 at the age of 85.

He was the son of Dr Thomas Cochrane, the famous missionary who founded the Union and Medical College in Peking. Robert Cochrane was born in China and was captured with the rest of his family trying to escape during the nineteen hundred Boxer Rising.

He was trained in Britain and went out to India in the mid 1920s with the Mission to Lepers. Later, for ten years he was the Director of the Madras Leprosy Campaign and Director of Research and combined these posts with being Principal of the Christian Medical College at Vellore, Professor of Medicine and Director of Rural Medicine. He converted CMCH from a women's college to a co-educational one and played a leading role in making it the outstanding Medical College in India. In 1935 he was awarded the Kaiser-i-Hind Medal for his outstanding work.

On his return to Britain he continued his work in the field of leprosy relief and research and pioneered the use of dapsone, still standard therapy. He was adviser on leprosy to the Ministry of Health and pioneered early diagnosis and persuaded surgeons to take an interest in the prevention and correction of deformities. He wrote textbooks, which became standard works on the subject.

After his retirement he continued his mission to lepers in Madras, as Medical Superintendent of the Leprosy Hospital at Vadathorasalur. Later he moved to a leprosarium in Tanzania.

It was said of him, "*A sincere practicing Christian, Dr Cochrane was equally at home in the pulpit and at the bedside*". Two of his children have also served in the mission field. Whilst at Vellore he was awarded the CMG medal by Britain and this is still kept safe at CMCH.

A Personal Memory

by Eirene M Mills

Dr Robert Cochrane or "*Bob*" as we affectionately knew him, was asked in 1944 by Dr Ida Scudder to be the first Principal of the Vellore Medical School which had to be upgraded to MBBS standard. His first task was to assemble and recruit a staff to fulfil University requirements by 1945: later he was appointed Director of CMCH.

I first met him in 1945 when he was in the UK and I remember how quickly he put me at ease by suggesting that we talk while walking along Hove promenade to buy some scarce bananas for a child.

Later when I arrived at Katpadi Station, he was there to meet me and for my first three weeks at CMCH I lived with him and Ivy in their small flat, as there was no other accommodation. This was typical of Bob and Ivy – their warmth and kindness and their willingness to share their home with a comparative stranger and a very junior member of the staff!

In spite of his greatness and excellence in the medical world, Bob was essentially a very humble man. He and Ivy were always supportive and helpful and both my husband and I owe Bob a great debt of gratitude. If it had not been for one of his many visits to our home on his way to see a patient in Poole, it is unlikely that we would have had our daughter. It was through his intervention that he arranged for me to see one of his friends, an eminent gynaecologist.

Bob had a strong faith and firmly believed in the guidance of God through his life. He used to carry some gospels in his car and when giving lifts to hitchhikers, always gave them a gospel when they reached their destination.

It has been a great privilege and joy to know Bob Cochrane and I treasure his memory.

THE RIGHT REVD LESSLIE NEWBIGIN

Lesslie Newbigin a Vice-President of the Friends of Vellore died on 30th January 1998. As the obituary in "*The Times*" said, "*He was one of the foremost missionary statesmen of his generation and an outstanding worker in the cause of Christian reunion*".

In his youth he was involved in the Student Christian Movement and after ordination, went to India as a missionary with his wife Helen. There he was elected to be one of the Bishops consecrated at the inauguration of the Church of South India in 1947.

The CSI sent him to the first Assembly of the World Council of Churches and in 1959 he left India to become General Secretary of the International Missionary Council, soon to be integrated with the World Council of Churches.

In 1965 he was recalled to South India as Bishop of Madras from which post he retired in 1974, travelling to England overland by bus.

He then became a lecturer in the theology of mission at Selly Oak Colleges, Birmingham for five years and from 1978-79 served as Moderator of the General Assembly of the United Reformed Church. He also spent 8 years as the part-time Minister of Winson Green URC.

Lesslie Newbigin was also well known as the author of many books, including the successful "The other side of 1984". This book especially lead to many invitations to lecture across the world and in 1997, he spoke at the Conference on World Mission and Evangelism in Brazil.

CH

James McGilvray CMCH 1944-1949

James McGilvray ("Mac") who died on 6th August 1993 was Bursar and Secretary to the Council at Vellore Christian Medical College and Hospital from 1944 to 1949, during the vital period when the College was being upgraded from the LRCS MRCP diploma for women to the full MBBS degree for both men and women. This involved meeting regular deadlines for affiliation to the University of Madras. The Hospital bed complement was increased during this time from 250 (women and children only) to 1,000 with all specialities being incorporated. There was an intensive and extensive building programme to provide the necessary accommodation, not only for extra Wards but also for departments of Pathology, Bacteriology, and Pharmacy, operating Theatres, etc., together with hostels and houses for the increased staff.

Mac was largely responsible for organising this and solving the many problems of administration. He was also involved in helping to organise appeals for funds and recruiting staff in the UK, USA, Canada, Australia and Europe. Vellore owes a great deal of his enthusiasm and energy during those early difficult years.

A Short Memoir of My Time in Vellore 1940s-1950s

by Paul Brand

I came to Vellore under a one year contract at the earnest insistence of Dr Robert Cochrane who was the first Principal of the Christian Medical College after it had been upgraded to University status. It was in 1945 and I had graduated at University College London Medical School and then took my FRCS in 1946. My wife, Dr Margaret and I felt sure that God wanted us to serve somewhere overseas as medical missionaries, but we did not know where. My mother, known as "Granny Brand", had worked all her life in the Salem district of South India and was a friend of Dr Ida Scudder and had followed the growth and then the upgrading of the Christian Medical College from being a LMP school for women only, until it was accepted by Madras University as being suitable for MBBS for 25 women and 10 men (in the first instance).

The university, in the person of Sir Laksmanaswami Mudalier, had determined that there must be a minimum of two surgeons with teaching qualifications before any students were admitted from Pre-Clinical to Clinical years. Two senior surgeons were indeed in place when the first seven students, all women, moved up from First MB and Pre Clinical studies into their first clinical year. However, soon afterwards one of the two surgeons (Dr McPherson) became seriously ill and had to be sent to England with the expectation of needing a year on furlough before he could return to India.

This was a crisis! The university commission was shortly coming to Vellore from Madras to inspect the school and if there was only one qualified surgeon on board as a teacher, the whole scheme might be disallowed. It was then that Dr Cochrane desperately sought for a possible substitute and it was then that my mother happened to be in Vellore and said to Dr Cochrane, "*You know my son is a surgeon. I think he would come if there was a*

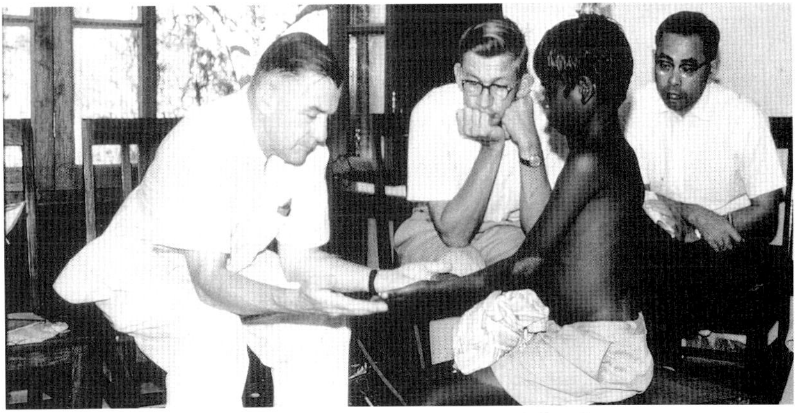

Dr Paul Brand examining patient's hands

serious need." Dr Cochrane said "*I'm sorry, but he would not do. We must have somebody with an FRCS or he wouldn't be recognized as a teacher.*" My mother proudly lifted her head saying "*But my son has just passed his FRCS.*" Dr Cochrane changed his tune and immediately sent a telegram asking me to meet him on Victoria Station under the clock on a certain date.

Margaret and I had one little son and she was pregnant with what was to be our first daughter. I was due to be called up into the army and the preliminary paperwork had already been done. However, there was no refusing Dr Cochrane. He went to the Central Medical War Committee and told them that I would be fulfiling a higher duty to the British Empire if I went to India to teach surgery than if I joined the army. He told Margaret that Vellore was a wonderful place to bring up children and she should follow me as soon as the baby was born.

So it came about that Dr Carman and I were the two recognized teachers of all the specialties of surgery, including anaesthesia and dentistry! Dr Carman was a very senior and experienced surgeon from America who had worked in India for years and I was looked upon as just a boy from England but I was good at bluffing and the students appreciated my style of teaching which included quite a bit of humour. I seemed to have a knack of imitating various types of disease and physical signs of disease and would often come into the lecture room limping in a certain way, or holding my hand over my stomach or my heart with an expression of face that was supposed to tell the students the nature of my pain. They had to guess the diagnosis.

I moved in as a guest of Dr and Mrs Carman and their family in a bungalow in Viruthempet. It was across the Palar River and a couple of miles from the hospital. One car was allocated to us two surgeons, an old Chevrolet number MDJ 693. I remember that car because it had no effective self-starter and could only be started by being pushed. Dr Carman and I took alternate nights to be on call for whenever serious cases were admitted during the night. We had no telephones and the only way we could be called was to send a peon on a bicycle with a hurricane lantern from the hospital across the river to Viruthempet. The peon would walk around the house throwing little stones up to the windows until one or other of us awakened. The one of us who was on call for that night would go to the hospital in MDJ 693 but the other one had to get up as well because whoever was not driving had to push the car to get it to start (with the help of the peon).

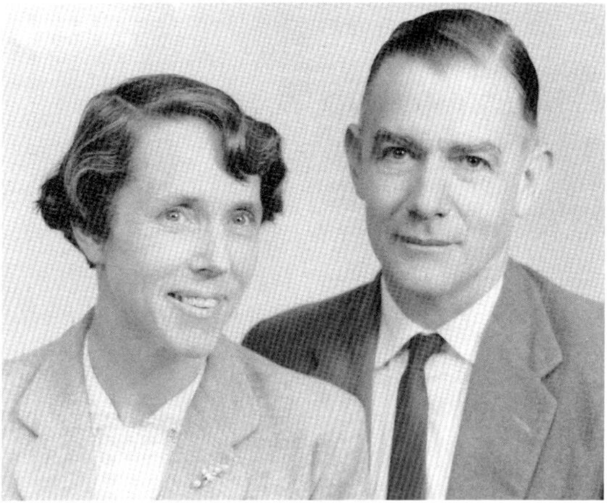

Margaret & Paul Brand, 1960

Over the next months and years other staff members began to arrive at Vellore. They came one by one from Britain and from the United States; from Australia and from other parts of India. Each one seemed to bring not only new strength but new requirements. There was Reeve Betts, the great thoracic surgeon from the Leahy Clinic in Boston, USA. He was the first fully qualified thoracic surgeon in all of India and he became the father of lung and heart surgery in all India, because it was his trainees from Vellore who filled the posts in the All India Institute and in other medical colleges. There was tremendous demand for his services when he first arrived but nobody had told Dr Betts that we had no blood bank at Vellore. He could not face the prospect of the kind of surgery he wanted to do without having blood available to compensate for the severe blood loss that may occur in these kinds of cases.

Dr Betts tackled this problem head-on with a dramatic plan that severely depleted his own personal blood supply but that finished up by making the need for a blood bank so obvious that it became a high priority. Dr Betts' plan was that whenever he had a serious case that absolutely demanded blood transfusion, he would call together the whole joint family of the patient and explain to them by interpretation how this young patient's life depended upon somebody giving blood and further explaining that to give just one unit of blood could harm nobody. He then asked for volunteers. There would be great discussion amongst the family who probably were deeply committed to helping their family member but who had never heard of blood transfusion and who were not fully convinced that they themselves would not be harmed by donating blood. Finally they might push forward a small, elderly woman and say that they would offer her blood. At this Dr Betts would look around at some of these strong young men who formed a part of the group, his face and his balding scalp would turn red as he berated them for not being willing to give of their strong young blood and being willing to offer blood from what they regarded as an expendable person!

At this point Reeve Betts would call on me and say, "Come on, Paul. These people do not care enough about their relative. I'm going to give my own blood and show them that at least I care!" I would then respond with a rebuke that the whole family could hear. I would say, "But Reeve, you gave your blood to Manikam last week and to Lakshmi the week before. There's no harm in giving once or twice, but you can't go on doing this every week." Then Reeve would insist that I went ahead. I knew that Reeve had group 'O' blood and was thus a 'universal donor'. But with exaggerated reluctance I would get a bottle and put a needle in his vein. The astonished family would watch in horror as they saw the great surgeon giving his own blood and they would watch as it streamed into the bottle. Nearly always the quick result was that the family would shout at him to stop and say that yes, they would provide a donor. I was very reluctant to participate in this frequent drama because I knew that sometimes no other donor would come forward and that even though most times Dr Betts gave only a few ounces of blood before he was stopped, nevertheless he was losing too much blood and I was really worried that he would become anaemic. It was not long, however before word got around that if the family did not find a donor, the great doctor himself would give his blood and this was enough to persuade them to find someone to give blood before it got to the point of Dr Betts actually having to donate.

There is no doubt that it was Dr Betts' frequent donations that speeded up the organization of the first proper blood bank at Vellore. I don't know whether those who presently manage the excellent blood bank at CMC realise that it was founded on the blood of Dr Reeves Betts. Perhaps it should be called by his name to commemorate that sacrificial history.

We surgeons who were new to India were surrounded with diseases that we had not seen before and which required investigation and research and yet our time was fully occupied with teaching and operating and taking care of the patients who had familiar conditions that we knew how to handle. What we needed was TIME for research. I myself was very involved with tuberculosis of the spine and of the hip; the management of poliomyelitis and of babies with club foot, when almost suddenly I became intensely aware of the crowds of severely deformed beggars who waited outside our hospital gates and also at railway stations and bus stops. Many of them were exposing great ulcers on their hands and feet to excite the pity of passers by. There were clouds of flies around the septic sores and my first thought had been of fear that some of those flies would carry the sepsis into our clean operating rooms and treatment areas in the hospital.

I had never seen deformities of this type in England and I couldn't understand why these people wouldn't come into the hospital to visit my clinics where we could study their problems and treat them along with patients with deformities caused by many different diseases and injuries.

When I made enquiries of local doctors they laughed at me and said, "*Oh, those are just lepers. They would never be allowed inside the hospital. People are so afraid of the disease that all the other patients would run away if they saw lepers in the outpatient department wards.*" I found later that this attitude was common all over India and that the only way in which people with leprosy (we don't call them 'lepers' today) could get treatment, was by going to some leprosy colony or camp where help would be available. Some of the first leprosy colonies had been started by Christian Missions but since there had been no effective treatment for leprosy, the colonies were chiefly places of refuge and support. We arrived in India at about the time Dapsone was first becoming available, and this drug seemed to be arresting the progress of the disease, though it was not a cure. Now this treatment was being offered at Government leprosy clinics as well as at Mission centres. The trouble was that medical treatment did not heal the ulcers or restore the paralysed muscles that caused the deformities.

The thing that turned my frustrated curiosity into an active programme of research was the fact that when Dr Ida retired and the Medical School at Vellore became a College, the person chosen to be the Director was Dr Robert Cochrane, who until then had been the Superintendent of a great leprosy colony 80 miles away at Chinglepet.

Dr Cochrane was one of the few highly qualified physicians who had devoted themselves to Leprosy work. He had worked for years to develop his leprosy colony, founded by a Scottish Mission, into a scientific research centre. He had become convinced, however, that the only way to develop a full understanding of the complex disease would be to work in collaboration with a medical College, where a whole range of qualified specialists would be able to study the disease in the context of their own special knowledge, without having to give up their continuing work with other diseases. "*By isolating the patients*" he used to say, "*we are isolating the doctors from the stimulus of advances in other aspects of medicine*". The possibility of developing such a collaboration had been one reason that he gladly grasped the opportunity of leadership at Vellore

Even Dr Cochrane did not believe that any big general hospital in India would begin to admit leprosy patients. What he hoped was that a leprosy mission would build a leprosy hospital very near to a medical college. Only then, he reasoned, would a whole team of experts be able to study the disease without giving up their primary interests.

He was delighted when I expressed my interest in this disease and he took me over to his leprosarium on the coast to introduce me to the patients and workers there. This started me on my long quest to discover why the germs of leprosy caused these ulcerations and paralysis of hands and feet. It was exciting work for me but it caused a real conflict of time because I could only see these patients by travelling for some hours to the coast where the patients were admitted. The problem was finally resolved when the director and the administration at CMC allowed me to designate one private room where I could keep leprosy patients, one or two at a time, under observation. At the same time a team of our technicians both from Vellore and from Chinglepet, began collecting data from hundreds of patients, beggars and all, about which muscles were paralysed and about the distribution of loss of sensation.

It was in that little ward at CMC Vellore and with the wonderful team of keen helpers, that we were able to demonstrate finally that it was not the germs of leprosy which caused the terrible ulcers and the "*falling off*" of fingers in this disease but the fact that the germs of leprosy attacked the nerves of pain and touch so that people with leprosy could not know when their hands and feet were in danger and could not defend themselves from burns and from thorns as they walked barefoot. Their wounds failed to heal, not because leprosy produced what had been called '*non-healing flesh*' but simply because patients did not take care of their injured parts because they could not feel them and would not even limp to help an ulcerated foot to heal.

It was this early leprosy work in a restricted part of one Ward of CMC that led finally to our first successful attempts at recontructive surgery and then to the opening of a whole Ward of leprosy patients (called the TATA ward, because it was a gift from the company that started AIR-INDIA) and then to the building of the New Life Village on the College campus, where leprosy patients could learn new trades so their new hands need not go back to begging.

Finally Dr Cochrane's dream of integration was fulfiled when The Leprosy Mission and the American Leprosy Mission jointly sponsored the building of the Schieffelin Leprosy Research and

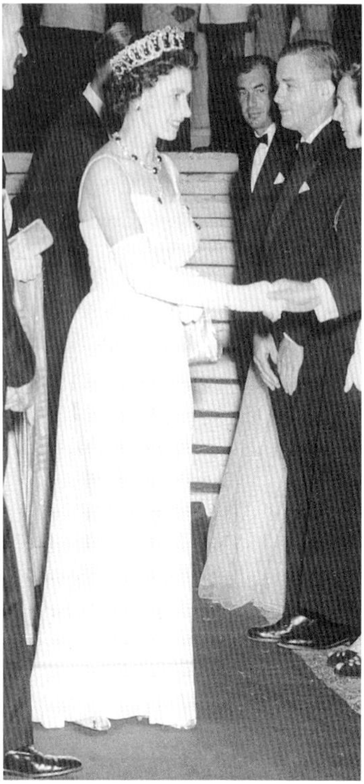

The Queen meets Paul & Margaret Brand in Madras, 1961

Training Centre at Karigiri, within bicycling distance of Vellore and the Medical College. From the beginning this was a collaborative enterprise with the Christian Medical College, with the agreement that senior teachers from either institution could hold joint appointments at both. This collaboration was sealed as dear Dr Ida Scudder overcame her physical frailty to come over to the Karigiri building site and hold the spade firmly and turn the first sod for its foundations.

Dr Ida Scudder, who had been the founder of the Hospital and Medical School, had become quite elderly by the time that we arrived in India and she felt that it was important for her to hand over all aspects of control to the new staff coming in, so I never saw her in the glory of her days of surgical achievement and leadership skills. However, she remained as a quiet inspiration to all the staff members and to the students. Dr Ida's snow white hair would be seen daily as she walked through all parts of the hospital. She never lost her interest in medical diagnosis and treatment methods. She would always ask the new young physicians and surgeons how they did this and why they did that and would always finish with expressions of admiration and even astonishment; then she would move on with her expressions of encouragement to help somebody else in another department.

The thing I remember most about her in those years was the frequency with which she would come into the operating room at the request of one of the patients. We would sometimes ask the patient what kind of anaesthetic they would like; should it be a local anaesthetic or a general? Many patients would just shake their heads and say they didn't understand about anaesthesia and they were happy to leave the choice to us, but they did have just one request: Please could they have Dr Ida Scudder sit beside them and hold their hand while they went to sleep under the anaesthetic? So we would call Dr Scudder at the appropriate time and she would come in with her gown, cap and mask and draw up a stool beside the patient's head and take hold of their hand.

She would sometimes pray with the patient and then encourage him or her to believe that the person giving the anaesthetic was a very skilled specialist and that she should be thankful for the great surgeon who was about to do the operation. I'm sure that all of us felt better and more confident with Dr Scudder sitting there and encouraging us all. I never kept statistics but I wouldn't be surprised to find that there was a better success rate in the surgical cases who went to sleep with that sense of confidence that Dr Scudder inspired.

Another vivid memory of Vellore is of the day that '*Aunt Ida*' died. She had gone up to the Nilgiri mountains to her retirement home and then word came by telegram saying that she had passed away. I don't know how word got around in Vellore, perhaps it was from the post office where they must have read the telegram, but within minutes it seems the entire town knew what had happened. There was no public announcement but quietly and deliberately all the shops began to close their shutters. The buses stopped running and it seemed as though the whole town quietly and reverently made their way walking to the great forecourt of the hospital. I have never seen anything quite so impressive as the unplanned tribute of love and of reverence by a whole town to an old lady and a foreigner at that, who had never had wealth or power but who had won their affection by the giving of herself. Many of the thousands who gathered were crying and others were telling each other of their previous experiences with Dr Scudder but most people had no words to say. There were no speeches. After a few hours the crowd quietly went home.

Something of the same thing happened when her body was brought down from the hills and the funeral procession led from the hospital to the cemetery. So many had gone ahead to the cemetery that it was almost impossible for the funeral procession to get in through the gates. The thing that impressed me was the silence, there was some sobbing and weeping but other than that everybody was quiet. She had lived her life in that town and that life had been an expression of love, the love of Jesus Christ from start to finish.

I personally had the great privilege of preaching the funeral sermon in the College Chapel a few days later, "*Moses my servant is dead … Now therefore arise! …*" It was an attempt to remind us that the real founder of the Christian Medical College was the Holy Spirit of God who had chosen for a time to work through Ida Scudder but now it was time not just to attempt to follow her example but to accept the Lordship and the inspiration of the same Holy Spirit who was willing to live in each of us to continue the expression of the same love that had motivated Ida Scudder.

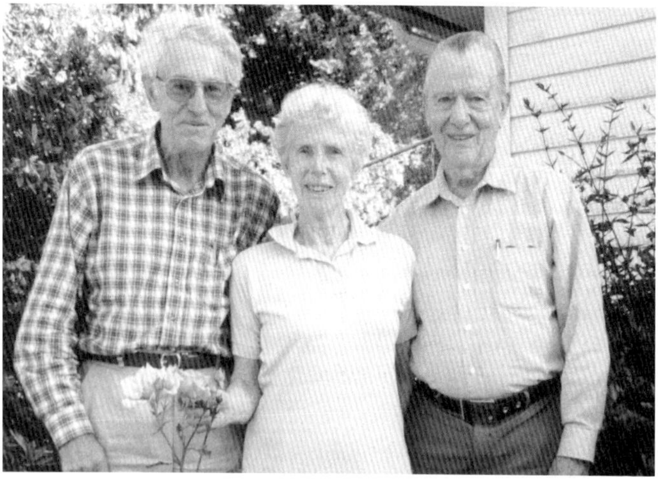

Jim Milledge, Margaret & Paul Brand, 1998

OUR EARLY YEARS IN VELLORE 1940s-1950s

by Margaret Brand

As I talk to young medical students today, I keep hearing about the major question in their lives, "*what should my specialty be?*" The matter dogs them for months, even years. I look back and realize that I had two days to consider the matter!

Paul joined CMCH, Vellore in November 1946. I followed when our new baby, Jean, was a few months old. After arriving in Vellore mid-year 1947, I was asked where I would like to work. We expected that everyone would be needed, filling in whatever gaps there were to complete our staffing needs. I had two small children to care for and could, therefore, be only a part time physician but was glad to help out wherever there was a "*gap*". Dr M D Graham was away getting further training, so her department, Pediatrics, had a "gap". That was my first job.

I soon realized that my experience in Britain, under war, conditions, was very different from what I encountered in Vellore. My two assistants were Licensed Medical Practitioners as were many of our assistant staff at that time. They did not have University recognized qualifications but had valuable experience and were very helpful. I also received generous support from the senior medical staff, to whom I often turned for advice such as, "what do you do for a child who has severe hook-worm infestation and only one gram of haemoglobin and you have no resources like a blood bank?" Then there were the children who came with severely damaged eyes but that was just incidental. They had more life-threatening problems. When those could be controlled, I would send a referral note to Schell Eye Hospital for them to sort out the eye pathology. I recall being very glad not to be on the receiving end of those referral slips! Medical training in war-torn Britain had not given me much preparation for a career in ophthalmology! So at the end of that year when staffing in 'C' Ward (then pediatrics) had improved and I was asked where next

I would like to help, I firmly answered, "I don't mind where you assign me as long as it isn't the eye department".

It was December 1948. Our third child, Mary, was two weeks old. Dr Carol Jamieson who had delivered her, was acting as Director of CMCH. The Director of Schell Eye Hospital was Dr Victor Rambo. He had been called away to help staff a mission hospital in Mungeli.

I was home on Friday afternoon with Christopher, Jean and baby Mary when a peon came to the house with a note from Dr Carol Jamieson. It read, "*we don't want to hurry you but we must have more help in the Eye Department.*" I wrote my response on the back of the slip. "*I don't mind being hurried but I know NOTHING about eyes. You'll have to find someone else*". But …. there was no "*someone else*", so within an hour back came the peon with another note. "*You'll learn. Please start on Monday*". Two whole days to think and pray about it. I surely prayed!

That Monday was a nightmare but we lived through it and somehow survived and even the patients survived the next few months. Part-time ophthalmologists working in private practice in Vellore gave us much needed help when their schedules allowed. I was grateful for all they patiently taught me. Also we had had a fine nursing staff, (Sister Sosamma was one outstanding person) and I owed them a great debt of gratitude but when Dr Rambo returned I was relieved to feel I was no longer needed there. I went to say goodbye to him. As we shook hands he looked intently at me and said. "*You have great hands for ophthalmology. I'm going to train you.*" And so began a wonderful residency in ophthalmology. Vellore's accredited programme for residents was to come later.

I look back and realize that I was just one of many people who had filled a gap when there was no one else available to do it and I was in the company of some great names, like Naomi Carman, Dr D L Graham and Dr Ted Gault, to mention a few!

It was some years later when I was able to help in the eye camps and could confidently do many of the cataract extractions, that I first encountered the eye problems of leprosy. Paul had already begun his journey into leprosy research, looking for answers to the mystery of leprosy deformity, of how to help patients get back to a worthwhile life when that disease had affected them but I was fully occupied with general ophthalmology and with being a mother! We did not see leprosy patients in our clinic at the Schell Eye Hospital so I knew nothing about it and was too busy with other things to get into the subject.

We had completed a busy eye camp in a village some miles from Vellore. The instruments and operating tables were being loaded onto the trailer as we looked over the many patients who, with eyes bandaged, lay quietly on their mats. My attention went to a little group of people standing apart from the crowd who had gathered around us. I asked one of the camp helpers "*Who are those people? They have come too late*". He glanced up, then answered, "*Oh those are just lepers*", and resumed his task. I wondered what his answer meant. Did he mean "*we don't know what to do for them*". Or did he mean, "*they aren't our responsibility, they should go to one of the leprosy hospitals.*" Or did he imply, "*they aren't that important*". I asked him to come with me and we went to look at the group. They didn't seem to be in distress but they obviously had severe eye problems and only one could see enough to be the leader of the group. They clung to each other for help. I had never seen anything like those eyes and had no idea why they looked as they did and what could be done to restore them. One thing I knew. I had to find some answers.

Dr Ebenezer Roy was Director of Schell Eye Hospital by this time. He was very encouraging and helped me to get started on my quest. We had one very small room designated for infectious diseases and into that little space we admitted a few patients so that I could begin to study the effects of leprosy on the eyes. I searched the literature for help and found some articles but the impressions left on me was a bit like the fable of the blind men describing an elephant. There was no consistent description or idea of when different aspects of eye involvement occurred once a person was infected by the mycobacterium leprae.

In 1953 Dr Ida Scudder turned the sod for the start of the Schieffelin Leprosy Research and Training Centre at Karigiri located about 14 miles from Vellore. In 1959 Dr Ernest Fritschi, then Director at Karigiri, invited me (one might say urged me) to begin studying the eyes of untreated leprosy patients. So, with the help of a recent graduate of CMCH, Vimila Chowdry, a wonderful assistant, funding from the Indian Council of Medical Research, and a splendid new slit-lamp corneal microscope donated by the Leprosy Mission, we started to examine the eyes (whether or not they had any eye symptoms) of the next five hundred patients who came to our out-patients department. When their time allowed, staff from the Schell Eye Hospital would come and join us. We needed their opinions as to what abnormalities were attributable to leprosy and what to other diseases. That help was most valuable.

So began my interest in ocular leprosy and interest that grew over the years until all other interests were put aside and I acquired something of a reputation as an authority in a previously neglected field and became an advocate for the numerous leprosy patients for whom blindness was the ultimate tragedy of their disease. Most blind people rely on their sense of touch to compensate for loss of sight. But leprosy steals "*touch*" too.

How glad I am that Dr Jamieson told me I would "*learn*" about eyes. And how glad we are that God gave us a wonderful opportunity to serve Him at CMCH, Vellore.

The 1950s

Radiologist at Vellore 1951-64

by Donald Paterson

In March 1951 I was fortunate to be transferred by the London Missionary Society from Hankow in China to Vellore. Very soon I had the pleasure of meeting Dr Ida B Scudder with whom I would be working, and Aunt Ida who took me up to her lovely bungalow in the Kodai Hills.

My job was to be Professor of Radiology and to take charge of the diagnostic side of the work while Dr Ida B specialized in Radiotherapy. At first there were only two diagnostic X-Ray rooms and the registration of patients was somehow done by Mr Lawrence in the dusty open courtyard outside the department. With the aid of Mr Vethanayagum, charge radiographer, I was able to establish a reporting office and soon with the grant of Colombo plan money, we were able to add two more X-Ray rooms and a proper registration and film filing office. I worked with Mr Rothschaffer to design and build the new extensions to the department.

My first excitement at Vellore was to make a trip to Delhi and Bareilly to try to set up centres for training Hospital Mechanics and Radio-graphers. While in Delhi I had the privilege of an inter-view with Raj Kumari Amrit Kaur, the Minister of Health, who helped me expedite the Colombo Plan aid for more X-Ray equipment.

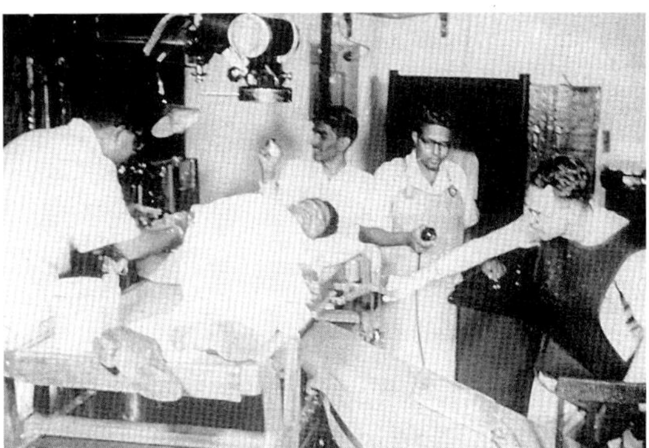

Donald Paterson at 1st Angiocardiogram at Vellore, 1955

For several years I worked single handed but with the help of Dr Ida B in the radio-diagnostic work. I did six barium meal and enema examinations and a lot of routine reporting each morning. In the afternoons I did bronchograms and other special procedures and more reporting. Most mornings at 8am I gave a lecture to the Radiographer students and for periods of ten days I showed medical students the workings of the X-Ray Department. Later I devised a series of 20 lectures on Radiology for the undergraduates integrated lecture course.

In 1952 I flew back to England to marry my long-time finance, Rachel Moore. Soon we were established in one section of the former men's hostel. Men students came to see us and marvelled at the neat and tidy home that Rachel had created from my old bachelor quarters.

Dr Jacob Chandy and Dr John Webb and families were our neighbours in those early days. Soon our son Edward was born and we had a splendid Christening party for him in the Chapel of the new men's hostel.

In 1954 I was due for a furlough and we had an exciting year in the UK. Our second son Andrew was born and I took six months' study leave in Liverpool and London. I got my MD by way of a Thesis on the Bone Changes in Leprosy but I failed my FFR as I did not have enough time to prepare for it. In 1955 I published an article on the Bone Changes in Leprosy in the Journal of the Faculty of Radiologists, London and later I wrote a chapter for Dr Cochrane's textbook of Leprosy.

In the years 1955-64, research became one of my chief interests. I was very glad to work with Dr Reeve Betts and Dr Gopinath in developing the first angiocardiographic unit in India. I was fortunate in working with Dr Selwyn Baker and Dr V I Mathan on the X-Ray appearances and function of the small intestine, and with Dr D M Hancock on the diagnosis of Bost Bulbar Ulcer. Later Dr A C Johnson and I specialized in the subject of Hiatus Hernia. Altogether I published 33 articles on these and allied subjects. It was the most productive period of my life.

My other chief interest was the work of the Christian Medical Association of India and I became the Secretary of the Central Board that organized the training of Laboratory Technicians, Pharmacists, Physiotherapists, etc. for the 300 Christian Hospitals in India. I helped to set up five training centres for Radio-graphers in different parts of India. I also became Secretary of the Church of South India's Central Medical Board, and tried to co-ordinate the work of its 57 Hospitals.

In 1956, the CMC persuaded the London Missionary Society to build a house for us in Vellore. In 1957 Somervell House was built just in time for our third son Alan to occupy it. Somervell House was completely enclosed by anti-mosquito screening, so some said it looked like a glorified meat safe! But we enjoyed it and were glad to bring up our family, of eventually four boys, in that pleasant place. A splendid tree house in the rear by the Peepul tree was one of the family delights.

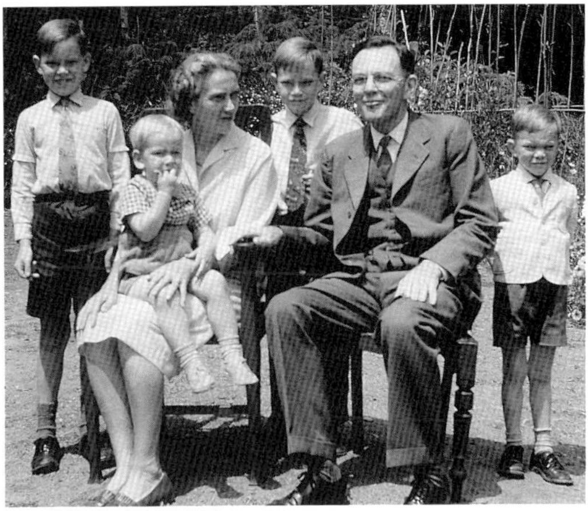

Donald Paterson and family, 1963

In 1961 Dr Paul Brand arranged for me to go to Hong Kong for two weeks to analyse the X-Rays of 840 Leprosy patients on the Island of Happy Healing there. Following this I was made a member of the WHO technical workshop on Leprosy and together we produced a WHO technical report.

In 1963 Dr A C Johnson returned from a two year period of study leave with his FFR qualification. By 1964 Dr Johnson was ready and able to take over the work of Professor of X-Ray diagnosis and I was able to persuade the authorities to undertake the much needed expansion of the department. With great regret I realized that my time at Vellore had come to an end and I resigned to take up the post of an ordinary Consultant Radiologist in Walsall, England.

1951 to 1964 were described by some people as the Golden Years in Vellore. Certainly they were the best years in my life. Since coming to New Zealand in 1974 I have been back to Vellore six times and now I am glad to be Chairman of the Friends of Vellore in New Zealand. Thus I am able to keep in touch with a really well equipped X-Ray Department and with the ever expanding life and work of the CMC Vellore.

A Dietitian in Vellore 1940s – 1950s

by Helen Butler (nee Witter)

I first went to Madras in 1946, having graduated in Physiology and with post-graduate Diplomas in Dietetics and Teaching. I lived initially with a senior missionary while starting to learn the Tamil language but during that time, with the help of my colleagues, I did a nutrition survey on families in the Bible School at Guindy, on the outskirts of Madras. I had been doing similar work in the wartime Ministry of Food in London. This was to prove invaluable in later years as I learnt the names and types of food used, their nutritional value, methods of cooking in the home and something of the customs relating to food. For most of four years, I was engaged in educational and village work, but had the opportunity of some part-time work in Physiology and Nutrition at the Women's Christian College in Madras.

Then in 1950 I was seconded to work in Vellore as Dietitian. This was a challenge in many ways, as some of the Indian Staff did not know what a dietitian should do and I was faced with adjusting dietary requirements for various medical conditions among patients of different religious and cultural backgrounds.

My base was the Hospital kitchen, Harriet's Cookhouse, with a small adjacent office. Harriet's Cookhouse had been built using money raised by Harriet, an American, selling her home-made cookies. There I had a staff of housekeeper, a clerk (both Christian), a peon (messenger) to do the heavy work and daily shopping and six cooks who were Hindus, a necessity for cooking food for Hindu patients. Repairs were often necessary to deter the predations of rats, mice, flies, cockroaches and white ants. Food was cooked on a 'chula' stove, a long low tunnel with holes for cooking pots and fed at one end by firewood.

The majority of patients had food brought in to them by relatives but the kitchen supplied free food for 59 patients and for as many other patients who were prepared to pay. A daily requisition was sent from each Ward from which was calculated the food issues to kitchen and Wards, the numbers of normal and special diets. Cooked food was taken to the Wards in large vessels carried on the cooks' heads.

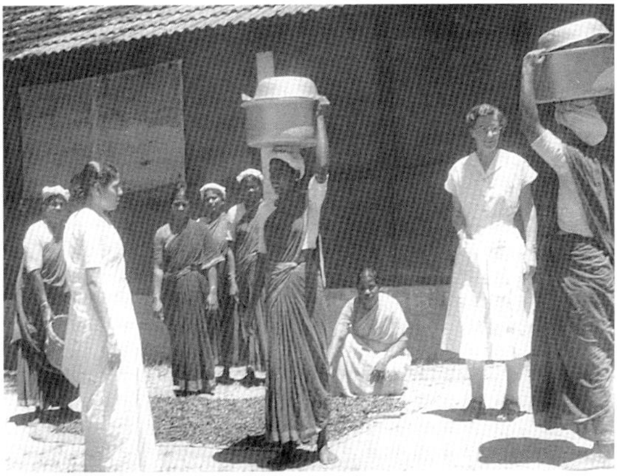

Helen Butler (neé Witten) with staff outside CMCH kitchen

Food for private patients was provided by a tray service from the YMCA canteen but I had to see the patients each morning and write out details of what was required.

I had only one year in Vellore to start with, but after furlough, dietetic work expanded considerably. I was asked to calculate special diets which could be used regularly for various conditions, mainly medical, rather than calculating on an ad hoc basis. While the principles of nutrition remain the same everywhere, I had to take into consideration the religious backgrounds, mainly Hindu, Muslim and Christian with some Sikhs and Jews and the relevant food customs of non vegetarian, vegetarian with eggs, vegetarian without eggs and European style and with alternatives to provide variation in the diet. Liquid and light diets were arranged for post-operative patients. After approval, the diets were published at the hospital's expense, as "*A Handbook of Diets for use in Hospitals in India*".

Difficulties arose when trying to persuade patients used to eating large quantities of rice, of the necessity of reducing the amount and cutting out sugar and sweet foods and the need to continue the special diet after discharge from hospital. Before Vitamin B12 was available as a supplement, anaemic patients were given scraped liver. High caste Hindus would take this as a medicine while in hospital but refused to prepare it at home. Sometimes strange conditions were encountered, as when a patient suffering from lead poisoning was found to be using lead cooking pots; another patient with persistent diarrhoea which did not respond to usual treatment was found, by taking a detailed diet history, to be using castor oil as cooking oil.

As and when required, I taught Diet Therapy to student nurses and student Sister Tutors. Lectures were given in the School of Nursing, but there were also Ward Teaching sessions when all aspects of treatment of one particular patient were dealt with in one week.

The scope of my teaching increased when, in each of two years, I had four students from the Women's Christian College in Madras, who had graduated in Nutrition and were studying for a Master's Degree in Institutional Management and Dietetics. They came to me for hospital internship as part of their courses. While they were being drilled in the hospital routine, they were also a great asset to my department, as between them they knew four Indian languages and were able to teach patients whose mother tongue was other than Tamil. When I left Vellore, one of these students was appointed to continue the dietary work.

I know that some time after I left Vellore a new kitchen was built. I was asked to plan such a kitchen and tried to do this based on a plan in an American catalogue, but modified for Indian requirements. I was not very pleased when told there was too much wasted space after trying to include all that was necessary! I do not know what plan was finally adopted or where on the campus it was built.

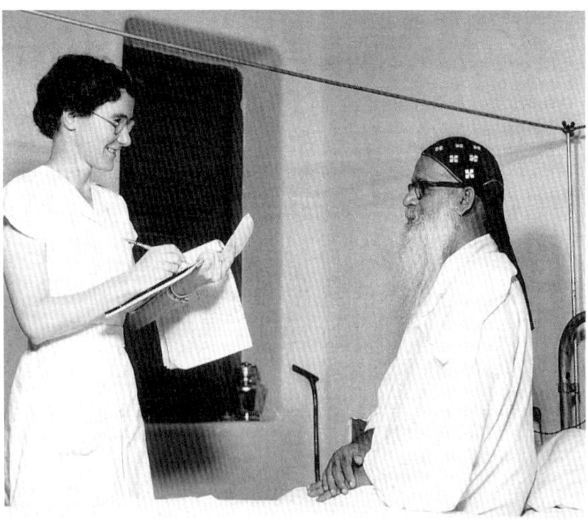

Helen Butler (née Witten) taking a diet order from a Mar Thomas Church Bishop

Albert Jefcoate: Vellore Concerts

by Roger Jefcoate, CBE Hon MA

David Chesterman's father, later Sir Clement, was formerly a medical missionary in the Congo and when he returned to live in Little Chalfont during the war, he became our family GP and encouraged Father to arrange charity concerts, initially for the Leprosy Mission and later FOV. I have many memories of the early Vellore concerts, many recitals in local churches like the Broadway Baptist church, Chesham which Father filled every time. That success encouraged him to try the much larger Beechen Grove Baptist church in Watford, which was equally successful. He persuaded many well known international soloists to perform for little or no charge including Nancy Evans (soprano), Beryl Kimber (violin), Alan Loveday (violin) and others.

Father then began to think the unthinkable and in 1951 tackled the daunting challenge of filling the Royal Albert Hall, something nobody had yet achieved for charity but with God's help those too were amazing successes with scores of special coaches arriving from considerable distances. Regular special guests included the Earl and Countess Mountbatten, Princess Alexandra, Princess Alice and other members of the Royal Family. Eileen Joyce was a special favourite; she became so enthusiastic about Vellore that she readily agreed when Father suggested a concert tour of India, including of course, a visit to Vellore itself.

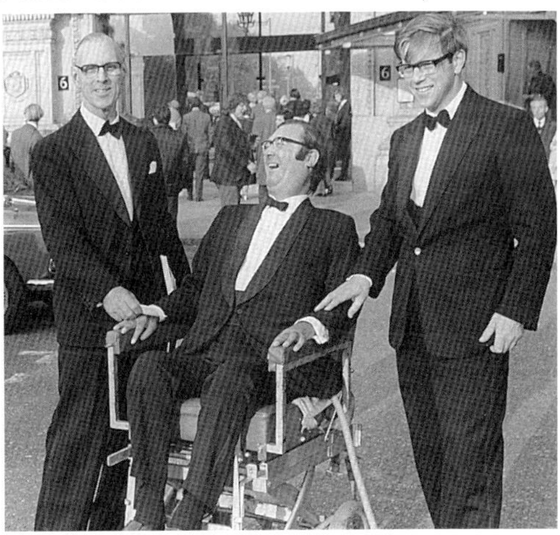
Jeff & Roger Jefcoate with a guest at the Royal Albert Hall

The 1963 Vellore

concert at the Royal Albert Hall was a particular highlight when I arranged for several breathing aid users (some on iron lungs) to attend, the first time anywhere that people with such severe disabilities visited a place of entertainment. John Prestwich (the world's longest lived iron lung user who still features in the Guinness Book of Records) often talks about those days when they came from their hospital beds in purpose built ambulances with police escorts: it was all very exciting and RAH staff laid on special power lines to the boxes and that became a regular part of these concerts for many years.

Roger Jefcoate has continued to help disabled people contribute to the community by using special technology. In 1998 he was awarded the CBE for services to disabled people.

ALBERT JEFCOATE, A VICE-PRESIDENT OF FOV

by Eric Gardner

Albert George Jefcoate, who will be remembered best for the Annual Vellore Concerts in the Royal Albert Hall, was called to Higher Service by his Lord on 31st December 1986.

Jef, as he was always known, was '*introduced to Vellore*' by Dr (later Sir Clement) Chesterman about 1940/41 when they both lived at Amersham. The Amersham branch of the Friends of Vellore was started soon after the meeting with Sir Clement.

Jef gave his fine organizing ability very generously to help Vellore. He had a wide circle of influential friends many of whom were persuaded to aid Vellore in various ways.

The first RAH Concert was given in March 1951. Eileen Joyce honoured us on no less than nine occasions, playing two concertos at each concert except in 1957 when she gave a recital. Sir Adrian Boult, Sir John Pritchard and Norman del Mar (nephew of Howard Somervell of Everest fame who was one time professor of Surgery at Vellore) were among the many conductors. At these concerts, arranged by Jef, all the conductors and artists gave their services for Vellore. Jef's aim was to raise money for and to publicise the fine work of the Christian Medical College and Hospital. Through the concerts many men and women of influence in medicine and commerce were introduced to Vellore.

By some, Jef will be remembered as one who 'opened doors'. Two examples must suffice. A letter from Vellore to the FOV office asked if there was any way to facilitate the import of essential equipment and supplies. Through Jef's friendship with Sir Cecil Wakely, FRCS (President of FOV) and Sir Frederick James (Managing Director of Tata Limited in the UK) a door was opened to the British Government. The Secretary of the Friends of Vellore was thus enabled to initiate and conclude negotiations which led to the Indo-UK Agreement. Vellore, along with all British charities working in India, thus benefited very greatly by the easy, quick and free entry of equipment and supplies.

Among members of staff at Vellore at that time, Jef developed a close friendship with Paul Brand whose leprosy research at Vellore is world famous. On his visits to this country in the early years, Jef opened many doors for meetings and professional contacts for Paul. They shared an interest in the production of promotional films and these were widely and successfully used by the Friends of Vellore.

Jef met Dorothy Clarke Wilson when she was in England to promote her book 'Dr Ida' and he suggested Paul Brand as a subject for another book: 'Ten Fingers for God'.

As one who knew Jef for well over thirty years, I can only say that God used a willing and industrious disciple to His glory. I remember Jef best for his generous ways, tireless energy and infectious enthusiasm.

MARGARET NASH AT CMCH 1948-1965

by Mrs E Mills

Margaret Nash died on November 28th 1993 in her 88th year. Following a fall she developed leukaemia and passed peacefully away prepared, as she said, "*to go home*". After a year in China, sent out by the USPG, she served at CMCH Vellore in the Department of Biochemistry between 1948 and 1965, and was for a time in charge of training laboratory technicians. The standards she set in her work helped establish Vellore's tradition of clinical excellence.

She was a gracious devout lady, a wonderful colleague and loyal friend, practicing her faith in a humble and practical way. After retiring to Stockport, she kept in touch with Vellore Alumni and for as long as possible, came to the Annual Reunion of the Friends of Vellore.

NIECE OPENS MARGARET NASH HALL

by Linnet Smith

When I was a teenager, my heroes were a lady called Ida Scudder who started a hospital for women in India, a doctor called Paul Brand who did wonderful operations on leprosy patients to give them a new life, an Indian doctor called Mary Verghese who operated from a wheelchair after being paralysed in an accident, the doctors and nurses who took care of a little boy called Thambi who was badly burned in the jaggery boiler and who told him stories of Jesus while he waited to be treated at Roadside – and my aunt, Margaret Nash who worked as a Clinical Biochemist at the Christian Medical College in Vellore. Imagine what it was like then, for me to be at Vellore…

…and to stay in Big Bungalow where Doctor Ida had lived, to listen in the Public Relations Office to her own voice telling the story of the "*Three Knocks in the Night*" which led to the start of it all, to handle some of her diaries preserved in the Archives, to climb College Hill and see from there the beautiful buildings which were the fulfilment of her vision and to visit her simple grave in the Protestant Cemetery.

...and to visit CMC Hospital with its 1400 beds and facilities like a MRI scanner, bone marrow transplant surgery, etc. etc. – and the ability to recharge my Video batteries as needed! To pray in the Chapel, so much the centre of hospital life and in the College Chapel. To visit the Ida Scudder ward at the Schell Hospital where free care is given to the urban poor. And to meet with a radiant faith, ready to share how God has blessed them.

... and to visit the New Life Centre and meet a man whose hands Dr Brand had operated in the early days – and failed – but who said to me, with a beaming smile, "Yes, the operation on my hands failed but from that the Doctor learned how to do it better for others – Praise the Lord". To visit Karigiri Hospital and to have made there a wonderful pair of sandals with the special micro-pore rubber used for preventing sores on the feet of leprosy patients.

... and to see sugar cane made into jaggery, to taste both the cane and the jaggery (just like eating demerara sugar!) and to visit villages with the CHAD and RUHSA programmes (the modern version of Roadside) so that I learned how health care is made available through regular clinics and how Dr Ida's vision of love and service in the name of Christ is being fulfiled today.

... and to visit the Mary Verghese Centre and see people with disabilities learning tailoring, carpentry and bicycle maintenance so that they could be independent and self supporting.

... and to see the Clinical Biochemistry Department with its ultra-modern equipment, reputation for reliable testing, enormous contribution to quality control in other hospitals throughout India and its wonderfully friendly staff including Dr Kanagasabapathy, who I fear has more grey hairs now, after the stress of looking after me for a fortnight!

... and to meet people who knew my aunt Margaret, those who remembered the Bible Studies she took with groups of students: those who remembered her as one of the "*old school*" of missionaries, prepared to work 24 hours a day and 365 days a year, those who, as interns, were a little careful about waking her in the middle of the night with a sample in case it turned out to be "*silly*" and earned them a well deserved rebuke: and one, a gentleman who was courting one of the young ladies in the Working Girls Hostel when Margaret was the Warden and who tried to avoid her as much as possible! To read again, in the Archives, reports of the Clinical Biochemistry Department, with my aunt's tiny neat signature on the bottom.

... and to have the enormous privilege of opening a study and research hall in memory of my aunt. The room, newly decorated, with its work benches and fridges and its small air conditioned annex for specialist equipment, provides working space for three members of staff and for the post graduate Clinical Biochemistry students. At the Opening Ceremony, Dr Poonoose Matthew prayed like this:

"*We are grateful to you for the privilege that you have given us to work in this institution founded in faith and built over the years through the untiring and dedicated work of a host of your children. Today we specially remember one such child of yours, Miss Margaret Nash, who gave leadership to this department of Clinical Biochemistry in its infancy. The seed which was sown by her has, by your grace grown into the present stature, as one of the most modern laboratories in this country. You have blessed us and brought us thus far and we pray for your continued blessings and guidance*".

It brought tears to my eyes, it made me so grateful for the prayers and influence of my Godmother-aunt in my own life and it made me so aware of how the seeds of Christian love planted at Vellore over the years have indeed grown and borne fruit in the form of a tremendous institution which is such a testimony to the power of the Gospel of Jesus Christ in that mainly Hindu land of India.

The Somervell Connection: Jim Somervell at CMCH 1954-1956

It was unusual in the early 1950s for a British doctor to join the junior medical staff at Vellore, to come to learn rather than to teach. For me it was a wonderful and revealing experience. When I arrived at Vellore in 1954 I was, as I had hoped and expected, thrown in at the deep end, joining a motivated and enthusiastic band of young surgical trainees, all of them Indians. From the first moments I was accepted and befriended, experiencing for the first of many times, the distinctively Indian genius for making a stranger feel at home, valued and accepted, a part of the family.

Vellore was my first experience of a Christian hospital. Previously I had been familiar with the idealism of British hospitals in the early days of the NHS but the Christian idealism of Vellore was of a different order. There was an element of struggle in it. The staff, and that included the junior staff, were acutely aware of the enormity of the health needs of the newly independent India and of the pathetic inadequacy of resources to meet those needs. There was a great sense of urgency to seek out the best ways of bringing modern, scientific medicine to bear upon the vast scenario of suffering. Vellore's Christian approach to this was (and I am sure still is) a very positive one. Disillusionment and pessimism did not figure at all, even among the junior staff, often inclined to cynicism in Britain but not at Vellore. There was a deep sense of purpose in their approach to their future professional work and it was in that context that we were friends and colleagues.

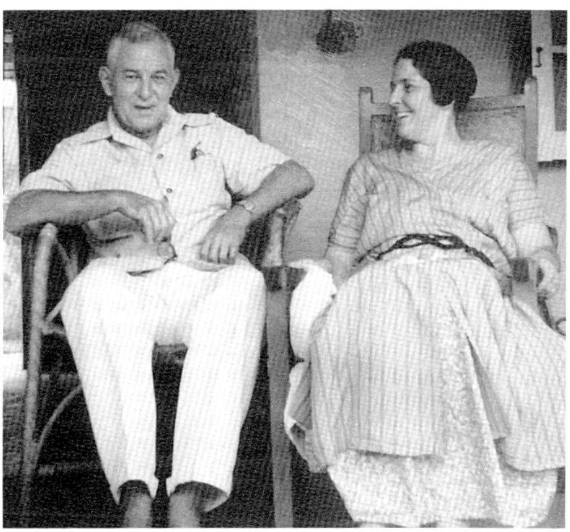

Dt T Howard and Margaret (Peg) Somervell

They were heady days, we were working in a rapidly expanding and developing modern hospital, linked to a newly-united Church (The Church of South India), in a newly independent India. The joy, for me, was to be part of this tumultuous environment alongside young Indian surgeons, as enthusiastic as I was. We shared confidences, hopes, fears and visions as friends together. What made this possible was the deep Christian commitment of the CMC and hospital staff at all levels and, I am convinced, the prayers of "Friends of Vellore" across the world.

That was in 1954. Since then Vellore has gone from strength to strength. Many of my junior staff colleagues of those days have contributed to this progress. In spite of progress, though, there remains the sense of the need of a formidable job to be done in India. This sense of need will be met today, as in the past, by a positive, constructive and Christian vision by Vellore. Of that we can be confident.

Jim Somervell was born in India (Kodaikanal) in 1927, son of T Howard Somervell and Margaret (Peg). THS was Professor in Surgery at Vellore from 1947-53. Jim was at Vellore in 1954-56 on the junior surgical staff and an Anatomy demonstrator.

Mary Somervell joined Jim at Vellore in 1955 with their two oldest children, Hugh and Sophie. Vellore alumni, who frequently were their baby-sitters, will remember them. Tom, their youngest son, was born in India in 1957 after they left Vellore to work in Jammalamadugu (AP).

Mary is now a Church of England priest, having been ordained in the first ordination of women priests in 1994 in the Lichfield Diocese. Jim is retired and a Lay Reader.

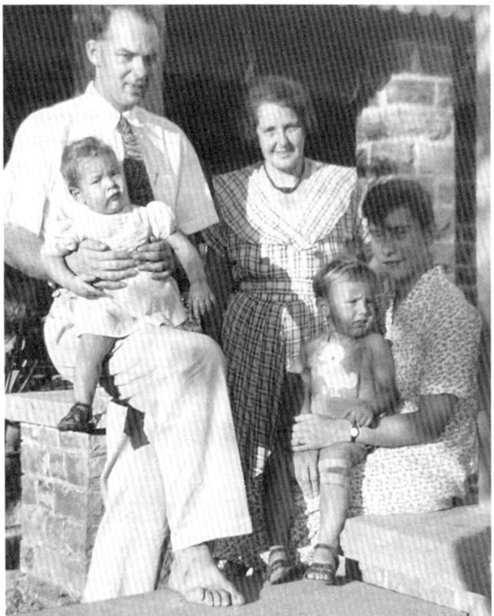

Jim and Mary Somervell and family

CMCH 1953 - 1971

by Professor John Webb

I first heard of the Christian Medical College and Hospital, Vellore in October 1951 when I was working as a registrar in the Department of Child Health in Newcastle-upon-Tyne.

Dr Frank Lake came to speak in the Medical School. I was deeply moved by his compelling account of the international medical college in south India and was immediately convinced that was where I should work. In due course Alison and I were accepted as missionaries of the Church Missionary Society and with our two small sons sailed for India. We arrived in Vellore in June 1953.

At that time Dr Ida Scudder, the Founder, had already been in retirement for some years, but she continued to live for much of each year in the 'Big Bungalow' on the College campus. Although she was only rarely present at formal functions and never interfered, her spirit pervaded the whole institution in a way one was immediately conscious of. I vividly recall my first meeting with her. It took place in the corridor leading to M Ward. She was coming away from the ward where she had just been visiting a number of patients. I was introduced to her as the newly arrived paediatrician from England. I do not remember what she said at that meeting, only its effect upon me. Up to then I had been a little uncertain of myself in relation to Vellore. Others had been kind and welcoming; everyone had shown warmth and friendliness. Nevertheless I was still a newcomer, uncertain of his ability to fit into this new and unfamiliar environment. But with Aunt Ida all uncertainty was dispelled. Her welcome was the most sincere and doubt-dispelling experience imaginable. One became immediately aware of the completeness of her commitment to the God-given task her work at Vellore represented and of her welcome, unhesitating and whole-hearted to oneself, to anyone, who came to join her in this task. One found oneself immediately totally accepted, part of her 'family' and with that acceptance, cautious

English reservation about the appropriateness of calling an unknown old lady '*Aunt*' vanished like morning mist in the sun. With that acceptance one was free, free to contribute all one was capable of and so one did and rejoiced to do so.

In 1953 CMC Hospital was already moving from a local district role to national recognition. Jacob Chandy was pioneering neurosurgery in India; Reeve Betts had introduced thoracic surgery and Paul Brand's reconstructive surgery had introduced a new dimension to the treatment of leprosy, which was gaining worldwide recognition. By comparison pediatrics was a very humble discipline. My clear responsibility was to develop a modern academic department. In 1953 the Department was recognized by Madras University only for undergraduate teaching. This continued to be the case until 1958. During those five years Dr M D Graham and I carried the responsibility for outpatients, a 30-bed ward and all the teaching. Teaching initially was based on western textbooks, which was all that was available. The diseases of Indian children had not been systematically studied and this we began to do. We developed a classified case records system, which enabled us to review our inpatient experience. This modest 'research' received a boost in 1956 when we invited the government Virus Research Centre, Poona, to study an epidemic of meningo-encephalitis in children living in the countryside around Vellore. The VCR identified Japanese B encephalitis virus as the cause of the epidemic, the first such identification in India and led to the establishing of a field laboratory at CMCH. In 1957 the first (Bombay) trained paediatrician, Dr Malati Jadhav, joined the Department, and in 1958 the Department was recognized for the 1-year training for the Diploma in Child Health. Although this involved substantial extra teaching, it also meant the presence in the Department of postgraduate trainees for one year at a time, and the enhanced level of patient care this ensured. In due course University recognition came for the MD, the highest post graduate qualification, and the goal of full academic status for the Department had been achieved.

One striking characteristic of Vellore was the uniquely close relationship that obtained between teaching staff and students. The first students had been Aunt Ida's '*family*'. She had not only taught them but had lavished all her care and affection on them. This established a tradition, which was very evident to me as a newcomer to the College. It was helped by the closeness of the student hostels to staff residences on the College campus and the ease of informal contact this facilitates. It was helped further by many formal structures; these included the final selection procedure for admission to the College, the staff-led Bible Study groups, student hostel entertainments reciprocated by staff entertainments and a staff-student cricket match (at the first of which I established an unsustainable reputation as a batsman by making a half century). This close relationship extended into clinical teaching so that the high standard of dedicated patient care shown by all Vellore staff was communicated by example as a norm of clinical practice, which a Vellore graduate could be relied on to maintain.

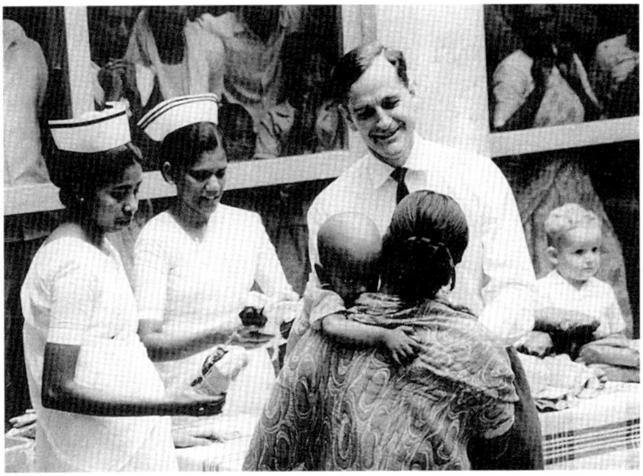

Dr J Webb distributing presents in the children's ward, Christmas 1966

One important strength of CMCH was the uniformly high quality of the clinical laboratory departments and their willingness to cooperate in clinical research. In 1957 the Paediatric and Pathology Departments embarked on a study of tropical eosinophilia, a common disease of the lungs for which the cause had long remained unknown. Ted Gault and CK Jacob undertook the huge task of searching microscope sections of tissues from children with the disease. Job's demonstration of filarial parasites in lung, liver and lymph nodes established filarial infection as the cause of the disease, which could be treated effectively with anti-filarial drugs.

From 1960 onwards a succession of UK trained Indian paediatricians brought strength to the Department, which reached its peak with the return of K.C. Mammen and Sheila Pereira. This strength found expression in the development of planned research in the major health problems of Indian children, malnutrition and diarrhoeal diseases. We liaised with the Central Food Technological Research Institute in studies of the role of vegetable protein in the treatment of Kwashiorkor and as a prophylactic dietary supplement for pre-school village children. We took part in an Indian Council of Medical Research multi centre study of diarrhoea in hospital admissions and in children in urban and rural communities. We liaised with the US Government Communicable Disease Centre (now the Centre for Disease Control) in establishing a Virus Laboratory at CMC headed initially by Dr Roger Feldman (of CDC), and subsequently directed so ably by Dr T Jacob John.

Looking back I see my first 10 years in Vellore as perhaps the happiest in my whole professional life. I had splendid colleagues to work with, nursing as well as medical. There was a marvellous sense of freedom as we worked not only to build a department but for the greater well being of Indian children. Paediatric departments were being developed throughout the country. I made many friends, some life long, among Indian paediatricians.

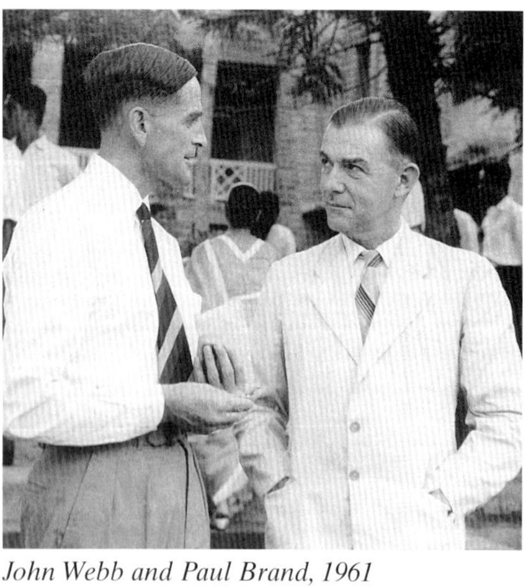

John Webb and Paul Brand, 1961

In 1963 I was asked to take on the wider responsibility of Deputy Director of the whole institution, I was initially reluctant to accept the partial withdrawal from pediatrics this involved. But gradually as I worked with the Director, Jack Carman, I came to recognize the vital importance of the job, and the privilege of working at the centre of this great institution. In 1967 when Jack retired, it seemed right for me to accept the invitation to serve as Director, even though this meant dividing the family with Alison returning to England to be with the children. It also meant total withdrawal from paediatrics but with the Department in the able hands of Malati Jadhav, Sheila Pereira and KC Mammen this was not a problem. My recollection of 8 years in administration is inevitably blurred but certain themes stand out.

One such theme was the growing realization that our undergraduate teaching was better suited to preparing doctors for sophisticated hospital based medicine than for serving the rural based majority population of India. With this in mind I suggested to Council that we should approach the Government of Madras to be given responsibility for providing the health services in a complete development Block, which would then serve as a teaching environment for students and interns. Council warmly endorsed this proposal in spite of the fact that it was bound to be expensive and no funds were available. Within 3 months Miss Julie Sharp, the Director at that time of Friends of Vellore, UK, received a request from an anonymous trust for a proposal for a community health project in India. A proposal was submitted, and resulted in a capital grant of £160,000 to be held in this country by a Trust, the income to be used in support of community health work. This in due course helped to fund the Rural Unit for Health and Social Affairs (RUHSA) in KV Kuppam Block, and continues to support community health work of the College.

Another theme was the need to modernise the administrative structure. This was brought home more sharply when the class 4 Workers Union suddenly went on strike, an extremely painful experience for which we were totally unprepared. The old pattern of benign autocracy had to change. A personnel officer, with experience in labour relations, had to be appointed and appropriate negotiating machinery developed. Changes at senior level were also needed. A selection committee to review staff promotions and appointments was formed. Senior non administrative staff were added to the Administrative Committee to help bridge the communication gap between administrators and other staff.

Another theme was finance. I well recall the tension in Committee when the Treasurer presented his Annual Report. Balancing the budget was always a desperately close run thing but we always seemed to manage. Year by year as the Institutation's running costs mounted, the proportion of income earned by the Instituation also grew. Income could be increased by a discreet upward revision of charges. A tight rein was kept on expenditure. This was facilitated by the provision to every department head of a monthly statement of his department's total income and expenditure, with a copy to the Director. That it was achieved without computers was a tribute to the organisation of the Treasurer's department. I was astonished to find in 1972 when I returned to work in the NHS teaching hospital in Newcastle that this essential information was simply not available.

Another theme was building. The major development in my time was the OPQ Block. This included new paediatric wards which the paediatric doctors and nurses had a major hand in designing. An important feature of the plan was the strict separation of infectious from non- infectious children. This meant the provision of separate toilet facilities for each sub ward. These had inevitably to be close to the ward beds: would such proximity be acceptable? Ann Sukumar, the departmental Sister, promised that an acceptable standard of cleanliness would be maintained at all times. I recall that I took the Chief Minister, Karunanidhi, specially to see the latrines explaining the rationale to him, on the occasion of his formal opening of OPQ Block.

An outstanding feature of Vellore has been the quality of its nursing. Vellore trained nurses were generally regarded as the best in India. I certainly appreciated their high quality on the children's ward. I was therefore particularly grateful for the opportunity I had of helping to resolve a problem that arose between the College of Nursing and the Nursing Service. The College staff were responsible for teaching nursing students on the wards but they carried no responsibility for patient care and ward administration. They wanted a part-time share in the nursing service. I chaired several long meetings with representatives of College and Service where the pros and cons were thoroughly debated. It was finally agreed that College staff should be accepted in a service role, an arrangement that came to work very well to their mutual satisfaction.

A vitally important aspect of the Director's responsibilities was the maintenance of communication with the overseas supporting groups. These constituted a huge international network, ranging from the strong and well established Vellore Board in New York and the Friends of Vellore in the UK to smaller groups built up round individual 'friends'. In all there were groups in the USA, Canada, the UK, Australia, New Zealand, Germany, the Netherlands and individuals in Sweden. Communication was best maintained through missionaries working in CMC but I visited all these countries on deputation, mostly on my own and one very happy tour of the USA and Canada with Alison. One found oneself speaking many times in the day, the groups varying from a cathedral congregation, or a university paediatric department to a class in a school. I tailored my talk to the audience but always I tried to convey a sense of the grandeur of the achievement that CMC represents. I truly believe it is and continues to be a great work of God. Dr Susheela Nayar recognized this. She asked to visit the College when she was the Government of India Health Minister. We organized a complete tour of the Hospital for her, including a visit to the Community Health Department. At the end of her visit as she was walking with me towards the old YMCA canteen for tea, she suddenly

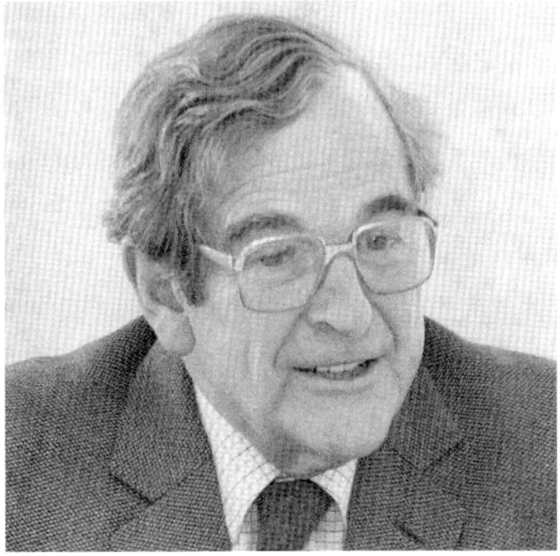

Prof. John Webb at the Friends of Vellore Board Meeting, 1983

stopped and said with great emphasis, "*Dr Webb, what I admire about Vellore is its spirit. I want this for my other medical colleges; can you tell me how to get it?*" I do not recall my exact reply. I appreciated her perceptiveness and wished I had the time to speak to her of the Spirit, which has sustained Vellore throughout its history.

John Webb left CMCH in 1971, Alison and their children having returned to the UK in 1967. In 1972 he was appointed to the Chair of Pediatrics at Newcastle University. After his retirement in the 1980s, John Webb became Chairman of the Friends of Vellore and for more than a decade contributed wise insights drawn from his many years of serving CMCH at the highest level. CH

MEMOIRS OF A WIFE, MOTHER, SCHOOL FOUNDER AND DOCTOR

by Alison Webb

When we went to the Christian Medical College and Hospital, Vellore, in 1953, everything was on a relatively small scale. There was a high proportion of foreign to Indian staff and CMCH was heavily dependent on overseas funding. It is a great tribute to the set aims of CMC, faithfully carried out through the years, that now the institution is financially self-sufficient, there are few overseas staff and this despite the fact that both Hospital and College have grown enormously. When we first arrived the College campus had large areas of wild and empty space. Some years ago when we revisited and I tried to explore at College, I got lost in the forest of trees and houses!

In 1953 Dr Ida Scudder, Aunt Ida, was still alive and her spirit was a real and enduring presence. Although she lived in her beloved house, Hilltop at Kodaikanal in the Palni Hills, she frequently visited CMC. She looked like a true fairy-tale grandmother with her lined but lovely face and shining smile, mass of white hair and above all, a keen and loving interest in everyone and everything. To my mind one of her greatest achievements was that when she retired she left this great institution, her 'baby' that she had loved and nurtured for 40 years and from then on, though deeply concerned and caring, she never criticised or interfered. How many people can or will do this? When she died the whole of Vellore went into mourning, a 'hartal' (suspension of all business) was declared and her funeral cortege stretched endlessly.

One of the pleasures of living at Vellore was the society made up of people from all over India, from many nations abroad and Christians of all the major denominations. Our Women's Fellowship (equivalent to the Mothers Union) at College was such that when each week one member spoke about her church, meetings for many months were taken care of. It was a wonderful environment in which to bring up children, who grew up to have no thought of colour or class and who sampled many different customs and cultures in the homes of their various friends. As a family we were introduced to Indian curries when, soon after we arrived, we went, as was the custom in those days, to the Men's Hostel for Sunday lunch. The temperature outside was hot enough to us, but inside my mouth was an inferno! At the end of the meal, my husband John was asked to "*say a few words*", another custom of the day. I was very relieved to be left silent, as I think I would have breathed fire rather than words! We all gradually got to love the hot food and became adept at eating with our fingers in the acceptable way.

My contact with the medical students was not great in the early years when our family was young. Later I was to get to know many of them very well, and they remain good friends to the present time. The girl students immediately struck one as graceful, lovely to look at and highly intelligent. In 1953 the men had only been admitted for the previous six years and one felt that they were still finding their '*identity*' in this previously all-women's college. The men too were extremely intelligent and very friendly and delightful. There was a pretty strict segregation of the sexes, partly imposed but mainly as the expression of the accepted social mores. There were of course boy and girlfriend attachments, and many of these couples remain happily married today.

One contact I had with students was in helping to produce plays. Each year there were several plays, usually of a light variety and the students acted theirs extremely well with a minimum of help from me. Two student functions were particularly lovely. One was Graduation Day, when the girls in double file, dressed in white saris with jasmine in their hair, each line carrying a vast jasmine chain on their shoulders, followed by the men in gowns and mortar boards, processed to the Assembly Hall, (later the Scudder Auditorium) for the presentation by a VIP of their diplomas. A wonderful sight. The other tradition was for the students, each with a lighted candle, to process round the College campus in the early hours of a November morning serenading each house with carols. (This had to be done in November as University exams were held in December.) We, and our children, thought this was a magical occasion.

Sunday evening services in the College Chapel were very special and I enjoyed singing in the choir, led by the Director, Dr Jack Carman. The circular Chapel, open to the cool of the evening and lighted softly, was a very peaceful atmosphere for worship. For Bible study, initially compulsory and later voluntary, the students were divided up into small groups and met once a week with a staff member. Latterly I had a group of girls whom I got to know well and became very fond of. Similarly in the College selection for admission process I was several times Group Observer for a group of about 10 girls, with whom one stayed closely for 48 hours as they went through a series of tests and interviews, (rather like the old Civil Service weekends). By the end, all of us were exhausted, but closely bonded as a group. The girls from my group who were successful in being selected for admission became good friends, and a source of 'baby-sitters' for the family.

One of the problems of working overseas is that of education for children. The local day schools in Vellore did not have a high reputation. So when we returned from furlough in 1958, our eldest son aged 8 had to go to a (far from happy) boarding school in the Nilgiri Hills 300 miles away. This we were not at all happy with. I consulted several of the mothers on the campus, Indian, American, Australian and English, who were either unhappy about local schooling or struggling to teach their children by correspondence courses. We decided to start a primary school – none of us with any educational training or experience! We had no building, no teacher, no money, few books, and 9 pupils aged 5 – 7. John and I offered our large open upstairs verandah as a schoolroom, we employed a young Indian teacher, Mrs Theodore, and Vidyalayam, the College school was born. One year later more children applied and we obtained permission from the Director to borrow money to build a small two-roomed schoolhouse.

Like Topsy the school grew and grew, more teachers joined, children from the hospital campus, (4 miles away) were bussed in, buildings mushroomed, and now there are some 250 children at Vidyalayam.

One of the teachers who came early on was the young daughter of very good American friends of ours, Prof Charlie and Betty Janeway. Their daughter Anne who had just finished her teacher training and worked for us for experience not for pay, which was fortuitous, joined us in 1959 and stayed for two years. Not only was she a born teacher, but she loved and was loved dearly by the children. The time came when the school was divided into three

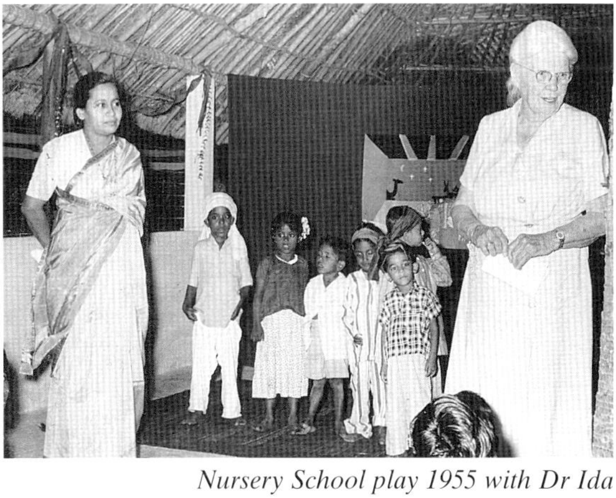

Nursery School play 1955 with Dr Ida

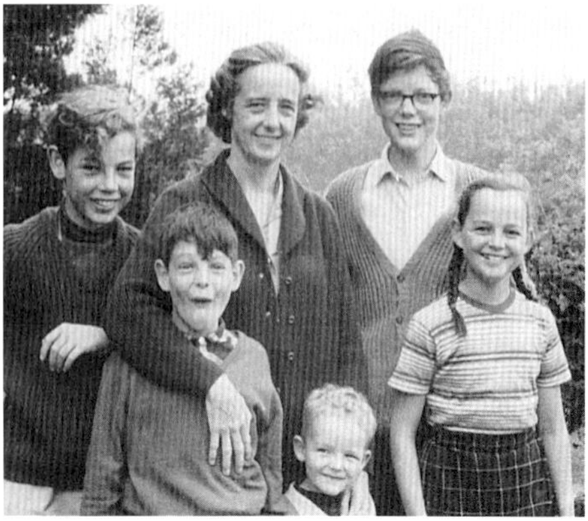
Dr Alison Webb and children, 1966

'Houses', and the children were asked to choose names of famous people for them. They chose Scudder, Lazarus and Janeway. And so it remains. Parents who wanted their children to learn subjects not on the curriculum had to teach them themselves. I (tried to) teach French, Latin and singing, with varying degrees of success.

As classes increased from Class 1 and 2 up to 5 and 6, our own Michael was able to return thankfully from boarding school. It is a very happy place, which was loved by all our children, and despite its present greater size, it has not lost the intimate caring atmosphere of its small beginnings. Lastly and importantly, the children do well when they move on to their varying secondary education.

Running the school from 1958 to '63 I did not have much time for medical work despite the help in the house of a cook and ayah. I worked briefly in different departments; microbiology, the antenatal clinic and the medical library. I started a child welfare clinic for the families of the lower echelon (and poorly paid) staff and in my last 3 years I began training in psychiatry at the Medical Health Centre. The CMCH had been built at College in a mango grove, a peaceful and beautiful setting for the mentally unwell. Each patient had a mini house with a room to sleep both patient and a relative, a kitchen and bathroom with a small veranda at the front. Thus they were cared for and cooked for (the latter very important) by someone close, not only comforting for him or her but a help to the nursing staff. In addition, the relative learned something about mental health care. As there were so few psychiatric units in India in the 1960s, we had patients coming from maybe hundreds of miles away and staying for long periods. The language problem was considerable but most of the time one or other member of staff could act as interpreter. I much enjoyed my short time at MHC and it led on to my finishing my psychiatric training when I returned to England for good in 1967.

During the hot months of April and May with our great friends, The Brands, we would go up to the Nilgiri Hills for our holidays. Margaret and I, she with 6 and I with 4 children, went first and the men joined us in May. We were offered the use of an unused tea estate bungalow in a village called Korakundah, 20 rough miles and a two hour drive from Ootacamund (Ooty), the main local hill station to which the train took us. In return Paul Brand and John gave a medical service to the tea estate hospital. It was an idyllic place, which we called Heaven, until the monsoon rains started. (Then we moved to Ooty and one year were offered a house to rent on Missionary Hill, spelt in the letter "Missionary Hell".) Korakundah was 6,000 ft up with perfect weather, beautiful mountainous countryside, rivers to fish in and picnic beside, lakes to swim in and panther, tiger and wild elephant not far away. Our fourth child was born while we were in Korakundah in 1956. The night before his birth, the Brand's aged and decrepit car sprung a leak in the petrol tank. There were no garages nearby and even in Ooty they would be shut at the weekend. So we plugged the hole with a sliver of wood from a gum tree held in place with chewing gum. That night I elected to go into labour and John had to drive me the 40 slow and bumpy miles to the nearest mission hospital at Kotagiri. With our guardian angels working overtime we arrived safely. While John and the very nice Danish lady doctor chatted happily, I produced our third son Philip a few hours later. This was the first (and last) time that John had been with me during labour – so different from fathers nowadays. Another memorable episode at Korakundah was when we poisoned ourselves with what we thought were mushrooms but clearly were not! Within a few minutes of the meal we began to feel ill. We had insisted, on the grounds of discipline, that the children eat some but mercifully they had only a little. Now we insisted that they (and we too of course) made ourselves sick to get rid of the poison as quickly as possible. The children suffered no ill effects, but Paul and I became giddy and disorientated and were driven off to the tea estate hospital. Fortunately by the time we got there we had recovered and needed no treatment apart from the kindness of beds from our friend the tea estate manager.

Our children were very happy at Vellore and had a wonderful free and open-air life, cycling or running barefoot around the 250 acre college campus. They kept very healthy on the whole, apart from the problem of septic abrasions on the skin when they fell over. Our second son Andrew broke his arm 4 times but that could hardly be blamed on the environment! Our daughter Clare, precious after two sons, nearly died as a small baby. Suspected meningitis aged 3 weeks, followed by prolonged gastroenteritis left her weighing 8 lbs. at 3 months. If John and his excellent paediatric staff had not been there to look after her, she would not have survived, like so many children in India in the old days.

Our youngest son Jonathan spent only 3 years of his childhood at Vellore, plus a 6 month visit aged 6 and I think he regrets this. But he has achieved fame on the rugby field later in life, which was something special for him and all of us.

These then are some of the moments and events that made up our lives at Vellore. There were more joys than sorrows, more going forward than going back, (though the latter was surely present), growth in experience and maturity and community, and hopefully growth in the spiritual dimension. My hope is that you will have obtained, in small measure, a picture of my and our children's life there and what a wonderful place is this Christian Medical College and Hospital, Vellore.

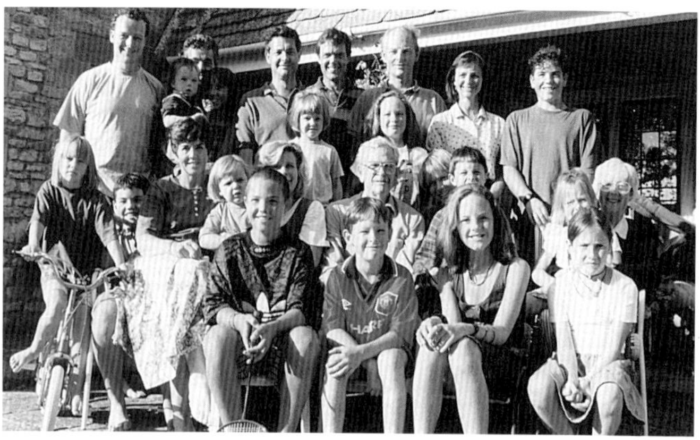

John and Alison Webb and family, 1995

MEMOIRS OF CMCH VELLORE 1958-1964

by the Lord Balfour of Burleigh, President of the Friends of Vellore

"*You wanted to meet John Webb from CMC at Vellore I think? Did you know he will be preaching in Fort St George on Sunday night?*"

I was told this by a friend not long after I had arrived in Madras in 1958, sent by the English Electric company to establish a factory for the manufacture of industrial electrical fusegear. My sister, a paediatrician, had worked with John Webb in Newcastle upon Tyne. So I went to Fort St George on Sunday night and had the opportunity of appraising a possible new friend by listening to his sermon. Needless to say, it was a good one, I knocked on the vestry door and was warmly welcomed by John who invited me to come and stay with his family in Vellore. It was the first of many visits in both directions between Vellore and my house in Madras, John would sometimes bring newcomers to CMC to breakfast with me in Madras and I recall welcoming Jim Milledge and his family on one such occasion.

The first impression for me on arrival at the hospital at Vellore was always the countless rows of bicycles shining in he sun, then, the long cool corridors with innumerable people walking to and fro, patients, nurses, doctors, carpenters, plumbers and patients, friends and relatives.

It was always fascinating to me to see the operation of the many departments. I saw the department of paediatricians grow. The practice of welcoming mothers to sleep by their sick children, speeded their understanding of what had to be done and assisting recovery after they had left hospital. Ward rounds, which I was occasionally invited to attend, were a delight. It seemed that patients, treated with great respect, often seemed to enjoy the attention of a crowd of bright young medical students. Laughter was not out of place in the discussions and students felt they could be bold in their diagnostic suggestions and manifestly learned fast.

Perhaps more than in most countries, practice was invigorated by the degree of exchange with doctors from other countries and by specialists with experience of new methods. The contrast for patients coming from the country where medical services were scanty into a hospital with international standards was always recognised and it was interesting ot watch the introduction of the carefully thought out Low Cost Effective Ward, which achieved important economies while preserving standards.

Passing from department to department along the verandah, one saw below on certain days a sea of blue aprons and uniforms billowing in the sun to dry. Back upstairs one encountered the large photograph of Ida Scuddder smiling encouragingly down upon the administrators. I had the privilege of being seated at lunch one day next to Ida Scudder and heard that firm voice talking with assurance and humour of the early days. "*Do you ever visit Kodaikanal*?" she asked me. "*Then you must go and visit Tree Tops, my house there*". I arrived on a day with mist winding damply through the trees, their tops invisible. After seeing around the house I was taken to the end of the garden where there was, over a precipitous drop and on clear days, a famous view over the plains. As we approached, the mist cleared, revealing a great area of south India, with hundred of twinkling lights in the growing dusk. Magical.

The siting of CMC among those hills and trees, lit by the early morning and evening sun had refreshed the spirit of many who have laboured hard there and remains one of the most abiding memories.

Many were the trips into the surrounding country to see villages, the oxen walking to and fro up and down a slope, dragging out of the wells a great rivetted cauldron of water which flooded down prepared channels to irrigate the rice in the surrounding paddy fields. A large tree was home to hundreds of flying foxes who would flap lazily around the tree and come in to land most skillfully, making an upward loop to grab with their feet a branch from which they would then hang, upside-down, ready to slip through the branches below when they wanted again to take to the air.

Quite early on I was summoned to a meeting with the Deputy Director Dr Paul Brand to see leprosy patients who had regained the use of their hands following an operation he had developed. They were making wooden toys. "*Could we not start a factory for these people and indeed all disabled people to work and allow them to earn a living again?*" asked Paul. Somewhat stunned, I retired to read a book Paul had given me by Viscardi who had done just that in America. With great help from Olaf Stroh, the Director of the Swedish Red Cross, a small factory was established at Katpadi, close to Vellore, employing only disable people apart from the driver and two or three in management. C Anthonysamy soon took charge and remains there today, 37 years later as managing director of Worth Trust, running now, four or five factories and many training institutes. Those trainees, in many cases extremely handicapped, passing out from these training institutes with a certificate obtain employment without difficulty. It has transformed the employment prospects for the handicapped in south India.

After I returned to work in Liverpool, I was asked to succeed Sir Clement Chesterman as President of the Friends of Vellore in Britain. A principal annual event was the Vellore concert at the Albert Hall. Many great singers gave performances free of charge and many great youth orchestras from all over Britain were a feature of these excellent concerts. Every year Princess Alice, our patron and a granddaughter of Queen Victoria, attended and Mr Charlton, the general manager of the Albert Hall, would have people standing by to rush out the red carpet when her Daimler appeared and roll it up again the moment she had passed. To the end she arrived full of life and, to the consternation of Mr Charlton, insisted on walking up a flight of stairs. She had always carefully read the programme so that when introduced to the principal musicians and conductor she invariably knew to whom she was talking and could talk of earlier occasions on which she had heard them. She welcomed those present from the FOV committee and wanted to know the latest news from Vellore. Asked on one occasion if it were true that her grandmother was as severe as reported, she said "*Good Heavens, No! We looked forward to her visits more than anything. She was full of fun, always laughing, played games with us and taught us a great deal*".

I look back on my visits to Vellore with great pleasure and affection. Apart from making many lasting friendships – (and acquiring the immense prestige of becoming godfather of Jonathan Webb, England's renowned Rugby full-back for so many years and who wasn't even born when I was there!) I regard the six years I spent in Madras as among the most important and enjoyable of my life and the opportunity to talk with the medical profession a very useful experience.

The story of the foundation of the Christian Medical College and Hospital at Vellore one hundred years ago is well known. But how many institutions started by a charismatic founder with such out-standing powers of leadership and inspiration have steadily expanded over a hundred years into a very large organisation indeed and have earned the distinction of the rating recently bestowed upon CMCH among all the teaching hospitals of India, while retaining the quality of the early days?

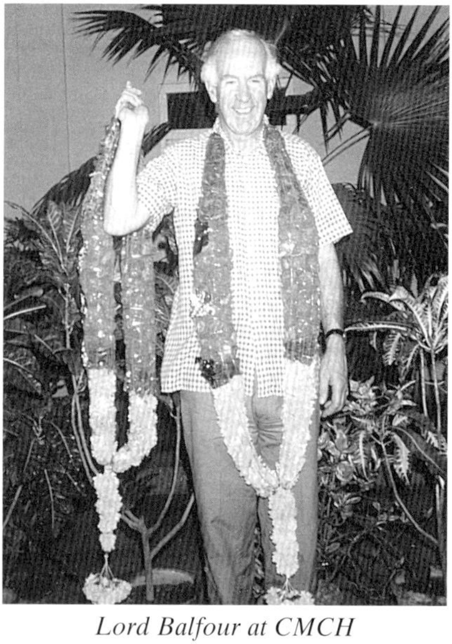

Lord Balfour at CMCH

The 1960s

Happy Days at CMCH as a Dietician: 1961-1969

by Ruth Angove

I was several weeks late arriving to take up my assignment as a dietician at CMCH in autumn 1961. We – 7 Methodist women missionaries and lots of others – had been seen off at Waterloo by Mrs Norman MacPherson (Mr MacPherson had been a surgeon at CMCH) and her daughter Helen on the boat train to Southampton on 15th September and on the way I had nearly died of peritonitis. I didn't die and so was unshipped from the Canton to a British Military hospital in Aden accompanied by one of the six – Dr Audrey Platt who was on her way to Medak CSI Hospital. After my surgery, I got a telegram from Dr John Carman, the Director of CMCH written in America, sending "good wishes STOP praying for your recovery". My stitches hurt with laughing and we stopped praying! We went on the next ship – Iberia – a month later and in due course Dr Brand drove me from Madras to Vellore on 9th November. He taught me that two safe and reliable drinks were coconut water and Brahmin coffee.

I lived on the first floor of the Big Bungalow in Hospital – where the Library now is. The rooms were horrendous – immensely high, colour washed with mustard wash, and my room had no windows – only three doors and a huge square hole facing onto the stairs. The verandah faced the "transport department" (soon to be run by Brain Witchalls), where there was always lots of revving, horning and banging the vehicles with various tools. I lived in 3 different rooms in that bungalow and my guests used to say they had never stayed in such a noisy place. I soon made friends and got used to the room – not to "bungalow life" though. The GS, Revd A Sanjeevi Savarirayan arranged for a small kitchen to be installed on our huge verandah and Agnes Forrest and I started "Flat life" instead – no butler for us! I always lived at Hospital, as did Agnes, even when we had our separate apartments – we felt that our friends lived there and that College was a place to go for days off. Hospitable friends at Bagayam made that a frequent option and we enjoyed the fresher air and the relative peace.

There was a lovely team of dieticians and their assistants – Rebekah Mani was in charge and Malini Chetty and Lalitha Venkatesh the seniors. Regina Sundararaj and I completed the dietetic team for that year, and the other staff were Mrs Mary James (Housekeeper – her husband worked in X-Ray), Mrs Vasantha Sunderraj (she was the Storekeeper and has retired in CMC Colony), Mrs Saro Finny Daniel and Miss Finlay Joy. Over my nine years Susan Koshy, Ahalia Nathaniel, Mary (Verghese) Mammen – currently Head of Department, Sarah Jacob – Deputy Head, another Mary Verghese, Lalitha Kalidas, Nirupa Roberts, Meheruneessa, Shanthi and probably others joined us for various periods. It was always a capable and strong team and I learned so much from all these good colleagues. I was sad to say farewell to all these friends though glad of the chance to put all I had learned from them to use when the time came to go to set up a Dietary Department in United Mission Medical Centre, Kathmandu, Nepal.

The dietary Department at CMCH was where the Wellcome or Williams Waterman Research block was later built. Access was past the "Small Bungalow", the entrance to "G" (children's) Ward and behind a fence covered with deep blue Morning Glory. Our Department was in "Harriet's Cookhouse" – there was a plaque on the wall to this effect. A lady from the Southern States of USA had been concerned about the lack of provision of food for the sick people in Dr Ida's Hospital – it was common to mission hospitals to save expenses on meals by leaving it to the patients' relatives (who are usually on the scene) to provide food acceptable to the caste. Harriet was unhappy about this and she made and sold cookies to fund the building of the "cookhouse". It was a brick building with a cement floor, the bulk of the upper half of the walls was fly-screened so that lots of air could get in. The roof was thatched with good access for rats and cockroaches. The end portion housed 6 tables and was our office. We kept detailed records, especially of the numbers of patients on free food – there was a government contribution to this and the records were essential – except when the rats got among them and used them for nesting. I made loud protests when I found a nest of baby rats eating papers in my desk drawer. The kitchen was a larger white washed area of course with a long wood-burning "chula" (stove), food cleaning and preparation areas.

Equipment included a large "attu kal" (iddly grinding stone) and another large "ammi" for grinding bulk spices. There was a Kelvinator fridge and a walk-in Blue Star cooler for storing perishables. When the voltage dropped, the cooler motor would groan and we rushed to switch it off until the voltage went up again. After some years trip switches were available and the motors cut out automatically, saving us some dashing about.

Breakfast and two main meals were served daily. Ward staff came to collect the breakfasts and afternoon drinks in "Basket Trolleys" – rather like small tin bathtubs on two wheels with a long handle for steering. Lunch and dinner were put up in tiffin carriers – five circular compartments fastened together in a tower with a label – and our staff took them to the wards on small two-decker trolleys. Trays were put in heated trolleys only for "M" (private) Wards at that time. After each main meal the floor was swilled down and the whole place kept very clean. I was therefore sorely offended when visitors who would look at the smoke stained walls and say "isn't it dirty?"

No one seemed to realise that a smokeless chula was not actually smokeless – this was very apparent when Harriets was demolished and another temporary kitchen of similar design was erected on the ground adjacent to "F" (thoracic) Ward. When we moved in and lit the fire the smoke belched upwards and the thoracic patients had coughing fits (not good!). "But", said the thoracic and administrative staff, "it's a smokeless chula!" Well, actually, the smoke goes up – into any higher building! The chimney was extended to take the smoke above the third floor and the chula roared away with a white heat like a blast furnace! Draught Control dampers were then installed. After a few years

Leco soft brown coal became available and this saved a lot of smoke and a lot of work checking the weights of the deliveries of firewood weighed out in Seers on a large balance at the back door!

There were always plans for a new pukka Dietary Department but although I stayed from 1961 to 1969, I just managed to attend the party when the Pongal was cooked for the builders – I don't remember if it was when the first sod was cut or when the foundations were completed. I did see the foundations in place before I moved on and I have visited several times since then over the intervening 30 years and I have always been impressed with the management, the staff and the products of the department. On my last visit we enjoyed a Christmas party and I was privileged to present the small Christmas gifts to the staff – quite a number had served nearly 40 years in the Department.

My strongest memories of CMCH are of the warm hospitality I received and of friendship and comradeship. Lots of the friendships have stood the test of time – I still get birthday greetings from some of my CMCH friends – and it was delightful to meet Ann Bothamley recently, as well as to be in a neighbouring congregation to St Peter's Church in Edinburgh, where Isaac Bhupalan was the curate – I remembered his father so well. Isaac and Amudha have now gone to Aberdeen. It is still a pleasure to meet Vellorians and hear the latest news and developments.

ENGINEERING AND PUBLIC RELATIONS 1962-1983

by Ann & Brian Witchalls

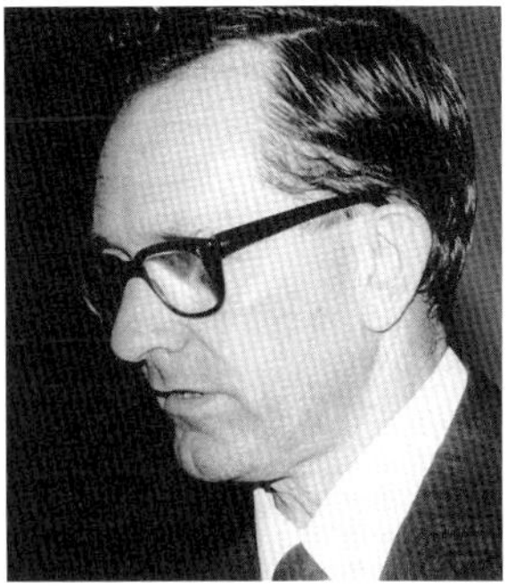

Brian Witchalls

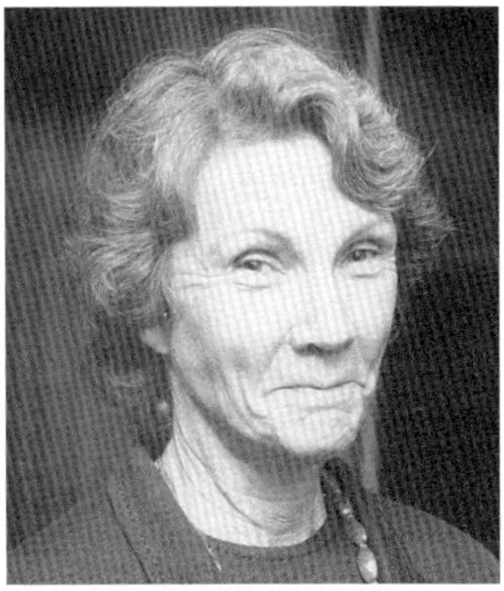

Ann Witchalls

Brian arrived in Vellore in September 1962 and was asked to take charge of the Transport Department. He started Tamil lessons with Mano Selvapandian, the wife of Dr A S Selvapandian, senior orthopaedic surgeon, (and with Transport Department staff!). When Ann arrived we continued Tamil lessons with Adi Kesavelu. Ann joined him in October 1963, carrying a fridge, wedding dress and wedding ring. We were married in St John's Church three weeks later. It was very much a CMC family affair. Ann was given away by Dr Selwyn Baker. Brian's best man was Thomas Joseph, the engineer brother of Dr Shantha Joseph and Dr Leela Varkey. The organ was played by Don Roberts. The College choir was conducted by Dr Paul Stephen. The ceremony was taken by the Revd Eugene Ten Brink, the presbyter of St John's Church. Ann had the use of Dr Mary Dumm's car and Brian arrived at church in Dr John Webb's car. Susie Koshi arranged the wedding reception in Big Bungalow. Dr Ida B Scudder kindly gave us the use of Hill Top. Dr Ida's bungalow in Kodaikanal for our honeymoon. We have written about this in some detail as it has been one of the few expatriate weddings at CMCH/St John's Church.

Our first son, Nigel, was born in the maternity unit at CMCH in 1965. This was the old maternity suite, even earlier than the present modifications, before the new Centenary Centre is built. Lu Carmen and Ann were both in the delivery suite at the same time, lying on one big table, with just a low, green curtain between them. There was great competition as to which baby would be born first. In the end Paul Carmen arrived before Nigel did!

Brian became more widely involved in engineering from 1966, setting up the first refrigeration section, accommodated in sheds. From about 1967 he was involved in projects such as the Williams Building, OPQ/engineering building, the present kitchen, laundry, CSSD and setting up EMD. He was in charge of College maintenance for some years, much involved with improvements to the College water supply. He was Deputy Director Superintendent (Engineering) for 6 years. We were in Vellore for the three month strike which took place at the Hospital.

Throughout our time in Vellore, Brian was a member of the College choir, and the choir of St John's which gathered to produce the annual St John's carol service. Over the years there were many memorable productions of the Messiah, Brahms Requiem, Joseph and his Technicoloured Dreamcoat and He lived the Good Life. Choir masters during the time we were there included Paul Stephen, Mary Oesterling, Bob Carmen and Poonoose Matthew.

We also got involved in other extra curricular activities: College Day, Hostel functions, and Staff entertainments. Ann produced many student plays and Brian was often roped in behind the scenes to help with microphones and staging. One memorable project was to build the illuminated caterpillar from Alice in Wonderland, sitting on a rotating toadstool on the pond in the sunken garden at College, for one Women's Hostel Day.

On one occasion at Hospital, Brian was on his way to the quadrangle in front of the nurses' hostel, carrying a plank of wood. He was asked what it was for. In answer, he put the plank on the ground with his foot on it, raised one end and released it. thus producing a large bang. It was to be the sound effect for a gunshot. Unfortunately, it was dusk and all the crows were starting to roost in the trees inside the Hospital compound. At the sound of the "*gun shot*" they had a severe attack of fright, so that the assembled audience covered their heads with their programmes to protect themselves from the fall out.

We took Bible Class for successive years of medical students. Bible class being the one subject on the timetable which was not actually compulsory. Before Ann arrived Brian did this on his own. That batch of students led him a merry dance, calling themselves by the name of other students and generally trying to confuse him. Many of them are still our best friends. In later years we also held a Sunday evening meeting to listen to recorded talks by the Revd David Pawson, an English Baptist minister. These had become very popular with the students when they were held in Peter Hill's house. At the height of their popularity we could have up to 70 people crammed into our living room and up our stairs to listen to the tapes. We always provided limejuice and homemade cakes as refreshments. These evenings were known amongst the students as the "*cake*" messages. We are not entirely sure whether it was the tapes or the cakes which drew the students! Occasionally we would be asked to host and to speak at the SCM Evangelical Students Union meetings after church on a Sunday morning.

Some years the Chaplain's Department arranged work camps for the students. The students would undertake a project at another Centre. One year it was to dig a well for a leprosy hospital at Vadatharasalur in Tamil Nadu. The students would work during the day and then there would be time for discussion and socialising in the evenings. These were always very profitable times.

Initially Ann helped in the Primary School on the College Campus for staff children. With no teacher training, she gave classes in French to two or three of the expatriate children, who did not want to learn an Indian language. She also taught Scripture. Then she moved on to work in the Public Relations Office at the Hospital, helping to produce the annual Facts and Figures, to write articles about the various departments and about some of the patients who came to the Hospital, for the Friends of Vellore in supporting countries. Two of the most memorable events were celebrating the silver jubilee of the Paediatric Department and the events surrounding the performance of the first kidney transplant operation. Two adjoining rooms in 'M' Ward were turned into as sterile a barrier nursing area as could be achieved. The operation itself was done through the evening and night, to keep the outside temperature as low as possible and to keep the danger from infection to a minimum. The Press had been alerted and we all waited eagcrly to hear that the operation had been successful , which it was.

CMCH has always been called "*one big family*". Sometimes those connected with the Institution have groaned at such an over used phrase. However, that is indeed what it is. One of the best illustrations of this was the active concern shown when Mrs Rebecca Mammen suffered uncontrollable bleeding following the birth of her third daughter. Staff queued up to donate blood and a round-the-clock prayer vigil was maintained until she was out of danger. This amply demonstrates the spirit, which is unique in CMCH – caring medical practice, under girded by Christian principles and practice.

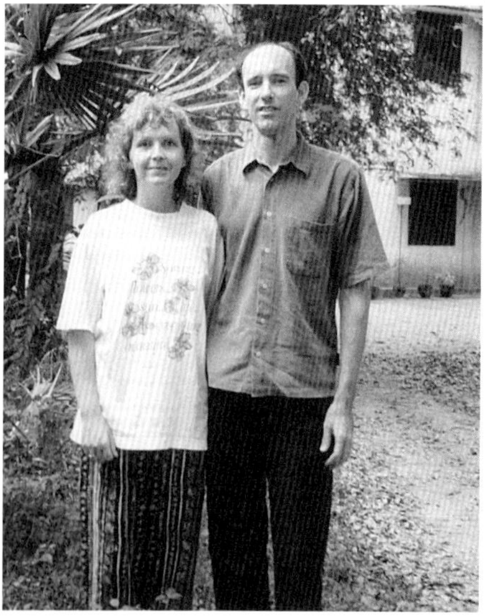

Mary & Nigel Witchalls

Ann and Brian's son Nigel, who was born at Vellore, has just returned with his wife Mary, from three years working in the Air Conditioning Department at CMCH.
CH

Dr Margaret Riddoch: Anaesthetist 1963-67

I have recently come across an account of my early impressions of Vellore, written in 1964 about eight months into my time there and what follows is roughly based on some of these early memories.

The Anaesthesia Department at CMCH Vellore, of which I was a member, had been started by the late Dr Gwenda Lewis and in 1964 two of her bright young Indian colleagues had recently returned from higher training overseas. One of these, Dr George Varkey, was by then Administrative Head of the department and Gwenda had a supportive role in the background for about eighteen months before she left Vellore, moving to Christchurch, New Zealand to continue her career in Anaesthesia. George Varkey was a tireless and vibrant team leader and one of my early comments refers to the good working relationship between the Anaesthesia Department and "*ALL the surgical staff, without exception*".

The theatre suite consisted of six operating rooms, only two of which (the cardiothoracic and neurosurgical) were fitted with air conditioning, which broke down each year in April under the strain of South Indian temperatures. The others were each equipped with several fans..... a world away from the sophisticated suite of 16 operating rooms which were built in the early 1970s.

In the 1960s, 450-500 operations were performed each month (excluding any under local anaesthetic given by the surgeons themselves) and as there were only five staff anaesthetists to cover the trainees, much of the teaching and lectures in preparation for their exams was done in the evenings, twice a week. In 1964, two or three candidates for the Diploma in Anaesthetics at Madras, joined the department twice a year and about one year later, we became recognised for training for the MD Anaesthetics.

When we were fully staffed (i.e. no senior anaesthetists on leave) it was possible for one of us to carry forward the "*Nuffield Project*". This was funded by a grant from the Nuffield Foundation to enable a CMCH anaesthetist to visit small

Christian hospitals and advise regarding anaesthesia equipment and whatever up-grading seemed appropriate in this area.

I was certainly struck in my first few weeks by the very small amounts of medication required to put our South Indian patients to sleep – in comparison with the UK – due in part to their poor state of nutrition and also often to the advanced stage of the disease for which they were having surgery.

At that time, ventilators were not in routine use in the operating theatre except for cardiothoric and neurosurgery – and I commented on how fortunate we were to have a respiratory physiologist, Dr Jim Milledge, available to assist with ward patients requiring mechanical respiratory assistance. He had recently designed and developed a "*Vellore Ventilato*r" (Mark I), which could pump air or oxygen into the lungs of such patients.

On the lighter side, I remarked on the custom then new to me ….. when any staff member has just become engaged or had a new addition to the family, he is expected to treat all his departmental colleagues to sweets or cakes. This practice is extended to a national level, so that when our Queen recently gave birth to her baby (Prince Edward), we British members of staff were forcibly reminded what was expected of us. We drew the line, however, at assuming responsibility for other royal babies born that year!

The wide range of countries represented on the CMCH staff and among medical visitors was one of the interesting and stimulating aspects of life which I specially appreciated; I recall a visiting thoracic surgeon from Outer Mongolia, who was very insistent that we should not confuse his country of origin with Inner Mongolia. Until then, I had not appreciated the marked difference which this represents.

I remain very grateful for the enrichment which belonging to the CMCH Vellore family has brought and continues to bring, to my life.

Dr Riddoch is a long standing member of the Scottish Branch of Friends of Vellore and is its representative on the FOV Board.

Reminiscences of a Physician at CMCH Vellore 1962-72

Dr Jim Milledge, Presently Chairman of Friends of Vellore

I had heard vaguely of Vellore as a great Medical Missionary Institution for some years before returning from a wonderful nine month long medical research expedition to the Himalayas in 1961. My wife, Betty, and I had an idea that we might work in the Far East in some capacity after serving two years in Hong Kong in the RAF. Then after the Expedition I felt that I ought to stay in academic medicine, that is in a teaching institution rather than in a small mission hospital. Jacob Chandy, who set up the first neuro-surgical unit in India at Vellore and was the Principal of CMC, was over in the UK and heard of us. We met under the clock at Victoria Station and he asked us, or more accurately commanded us, to come to Vellore. I was a general physician with a special interest in chest medicine and Betty was an anaesthetist. Both skills, he said, were needed at Vellore. The Missionary Society with which we had been having talks, the Council of World Mission (formerly London Missionary Society) were willing to send us to Vellore. They were already supporting Donald, a radiologist, and Rachel Paterson at Vellore, and so in April 1962 we sailed out to Bombay and then made our way by train to Vellore.

We had a very gentle introduction to life in India and Vellore with Don and Rachel to guide us. Our time in Hong Kong meant that we were to a degree acclimatised and of course Vellore, even then, was relatively civilized compared with the situation of many missionaries in India.

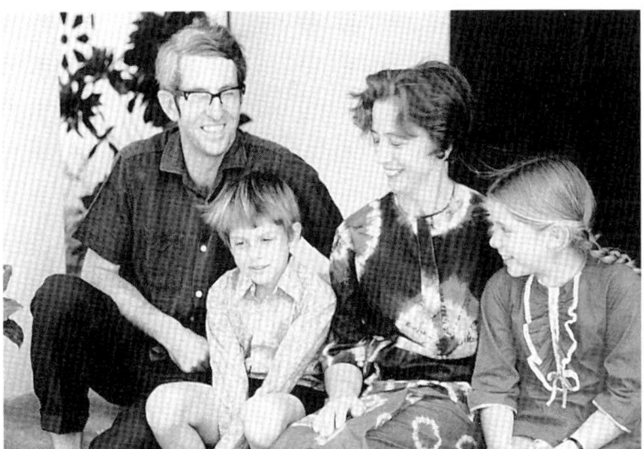

The Milledge family, 1972

My parents were working in Kerala and five years before we had visited them for Christmas and we had spent nine months in Nepal where Betty had worked in Shata Bhawan Hospital.

Our first home in Vellore was the "Quadraplex" building across the dry ditch from the rural hospital. The four units consisted of two flats and two corridors of rooms for Rural Hospital Junior Staff. We had the ground floor flat which was good, as the next year our daughter, Margaret, was born and her pram lived under the stairs. At first we both worked part time and had time for Tamil language study with Mrs Sevapandian, the wife of the head of Orthopaedics. Betty was better at the language than I but that is not saying much! The fact that one can get by pretty well in English does not give the same incentive to master the language as in more rural settings. The work of the College and Hospital is conducted in English since staff and students come from many language areas of India and half the patients are non-Tamil speaking. However, it was rather a blow when after I thought I had got some fluency and was talking away in Tamil to a patient he turned to a nurse and said, "*English theriadu*", - "*I don't understand English*"!

During my time at Vellore I worked closely with the Cardio-Thoracic Unit. I set up a lung function laboratory up near 'F' Ward, the Cardio-Thoracic ward. The Thoracic Unit had been started by an American, Dr Reeve Betts, a few years before. He had left and Dr Gopinarth, a trainee of Betts, was head of the Unit when I arrived. He was just embarking on open-heart surgery, working on dogs to perfect his technique. With my experience in cardio-respiratory physiology I was able to help with this work. It was hard and discouraging work with more failures than successes. This was true in units all over the world but we had rather poorer facilities than most.

There were no reputable dealers from which to get our dogs for this work and in one batch, one of the dogs became rabid. Fortunately no one was bitten but we had already used some dogs from the batch who could have been incubating rabies. So we could not be sure that we had not become infected from the saliva of any of these dogs. Therefore all of us in the team had to have the standard course of injections into our abdominal wall muscles. However, it was exciting to be working at the "leading edge" of surgery and eventually we were able to start open-heart surgery on patients. We operated mainly on young people and children with congenital heart defects. I helped with the heart and lung pump at first, much of it home made in the early days. Soon the very good pump technicians, Samson and Amalraj, became expert and did not need my help. After such surgery, patients need a lot of care in the Intensive Therapy Unit and as we were short of anaesthetists, I helped with the ventilator treatment of these patients. Another area where we used artificial ventilation was in the treatment of severe tetanus. Ventilators were expensive, had to be imported and were not very reliable in those days. I spent some time inventing a very simple ventilator which was eventually manufactured as the "*Vellore Ventilator*" though it was soon superseded.

We used to have surgeons come to the unit for a two year residency training in Cardio-Thoracic surgery and many of these became firm friends as well as providing an important component of the staff. Dr Bhati was with us when Margaret was born and in congratulating me said, "*She was assembled in India from British parts*", a reference to the way cars used to come from Britain in "*knock down*" form, and were assembled in India. Later Dr Jasper McPhail and then Dr "*Bud*" Wilson, both Thoracic surgeons from the States came to the Unit and finally Dr Stanley John, a Vellore graduate returning from overseas training, became head of the unit for the later years of my time there.

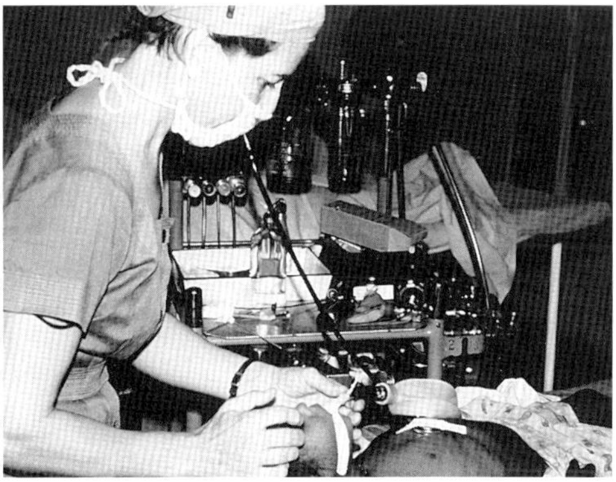

Dr Betty Milledge anaesthetising a patient, 1971

I also worked in respiratory medicine,

seeing patients with various lung diseases including tropical eosinophilia, an asthma-like illness, which John Webb and others at Vellore had shown to be due to microfilaria. We started a TB clinic using drugs supplied by WHO via the Indian Government. The problem was that the supply was erratic. We started using a fully supervised twice-weekly regime which I see is now being advised again for developing countries. For a very happy two years I was in charge of a General Medical unit (Med II) while Dr T S Koshi was abroad and enjoyed the work and especially the under and post graduate teaching. Lilly John (nee Thomas, wife of Stanley John) and VX Mathews were my colleagues in the unit. Also for a while I did some teaching in the Physiology Department under Dr P Zachariah.

Betty worked in the Anaesthetic Department, first under Dr Gwenda Lewis, then Dr George Varkey, and finally Dr Val Major. She enjoyed this and with her Nepal experience was able to teach, especially the simpler forms of anaesthesia using ether and simple apparatus, which would be available in small rural hospitals where many of our graduates would work. She also made a number of trips to such hospitals to help teach their staff newer, but appropriate, anaesthetic techniques.

We were both keen on the idea of promoting simple medicine where appropriate and partly with this idea in mind, when our second child was due, Betty decided to be delivered in the newly opened unit at the Rural Hospital. We went down there one evening as she went into labour and the Midwife opened up the place – we were the only customers. John was safely born in the night. The Midwife then announced that she was off and where was our Ayah? The village woman would, of course, have come in with Granny or Aunty or a servant. It was too late to get anyone else so I had to stay but there was no one to look after Margaret, so she was fetched and we all bedded down. All went well, though Margaret and I were covered with mosquito bites in the morning.

It was not all work at Vellore. Tennis on Saturday afternoons on the court by Big Bungalow with staff and occasional students was a good relaxation if it was not too hot.

Trips to Amerdi, Mahabalipuram and other beauty spots, swimming at Kadagiri were all enjoyed with our children. I was also able to get some rock climbing around Vellore. Mostly the rock in South India is disappointing in that, with no frost to shatter it, it is very smooth. So, if the angle is not too high, one can just walk up; if a bit higher, it is just impossible. However, we did find some places where there were cracks or chimneys and we played around on these. But the best place was undoubtedly Nagari. About 60 miles north of Vellore was this small mission hospital which became associated with CMC. About three to four hours' walk from it was a splendid escarpment four to eight hundred feet high, ending in a fine nose, reminiscent of General de Gaul lying on his back. With John Girling, a prosthetics engineer and later Graham Morritt, a medical student and others, I had a number of great weekends on this extensive rock area.

Although there were cinemas, there was no TV and it was mostly a matter of making our own entertainments. We did a lot of visiting each others' homes; sometimes life on the Hospital or College Campuses seemed to be a social whirl. Then there were student entertainments, men's and women's hostel days and plays put on by students. Once a year there was a "*Staff Entertainment*". Two that stand out in my mind were the "*Circus*" held on the Big Bungalow tennis court (George Varkey a wonderful "*Strong Man*" and Brian Witchalls as a clown) and the last one I was in, "The Batsman's Bride", a respectful take off of Gilbert and Sullivan, based of course on Cricket. Albert Paintal, a junior Doctor was the Village Batsman and Brian Witchalls was Old Willum the Umpire but we had to borrow a student to play the bride, Tulsna Rustomji a delightful, petite Parsee girl.

Holidays in Kodi or the Nilgiris are important memories for our family but are not part of these reminiscences, nor are the three trips I was able to make to the Nepal Himalayas from Vellore, nor the year we had in San Francisco in the middle of our ten years at CMC when I was a Research Fellow.

When we returned for our second term at Vellore we moved into the Webb's house and for about six months kept house for the

Director, John Webb. This was a very happy time though a busy one, with even more visitors then we had had previously. Indeed houseguests were very much a part of life and the job at Vellore. There were official ones, especially at Council time, through to missionary colleagues, often coming as patients to the hospital or to attend courses or meetings. This contributed to the richness of life at CMC.

Sundays were almost as busy as week days. We would all go down from the College Campus to the fort in Vellore to St John's Church. There we had excellent services led by Dr Eugene Ten Brink in the early days and later by the Revd Peter Bishop. The children would have Sunday School, coming into part of the service. I remember John, abetted by his friends such as Paul Carmen, would frequently be less than well behaved. After a particularly exasperating episode when Betty had almost lost her temper with him, the next hymn was announced and we could hardly keep a straight face. It was, "Can a mother's tender care, cease towards the child she bare. Yes, she may forgetful be .." Then we might go to the Men's or Women's hostel for lunch. The children particularly liked that, as they were always made a fuss of by the students and loved the chicken curry. In the evening we went to the College Chapel where I sang in the choir. The Chapel was so simple with its cool marble floor and flower decorations, The whole atmosphere of those evenings with the scent of the frangipani wafting in and the light fading was quite wonderful.

But the most abiding memories of Vellore are of the friends, staff, students and others who made up the community of Vellore. Whether Christian, Hindu, Moslem or Parsee one had a sense that they all subscribed to the vision of service that was summed up in the College motto. Not that we all lived up to this all the time, far from it but the ideal was there and accepted and yet this was not some freakish cult commune but a very busy, huge, working medical institution with standards as high as anywhere in the world. I count myself supremely fortunate to have been for ten years part of the Vellore CMCH family.

Looking In From the Outside 1964-1971

by The Revd. Dr Peter Bishop

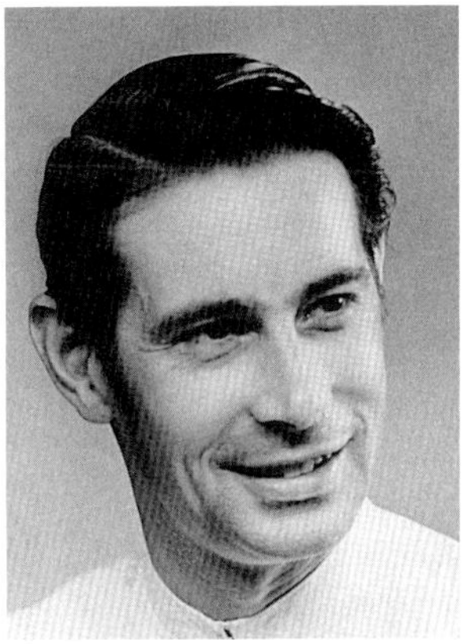

Revd Dr Peter Bishop, 1966

It was a different world. Not for us the instant transfer from one continent to another by aircraft. On 28th September 1964 my wife Anne, Mark (aged two) and I left Southampton aboard the P & O liner Chusan, bound for Bombay and service in the Church of South India.

Vellore was not in our thoughts. Unlike every other expatriate in Vellore when we were there, we were not staff of the Hospital or Medical College, nor did we have any kind of medical, nursing or paramedical training. A probationary Methodist Minister going to be ordained in the Church of South India and a teacher whose role was so ill-defined as to prompt her to describe herself on one official form as 'accompanying baggage', ours was a journey into the unknown. We had no idea where we would be stationed once we arrived in India, other than that it would be in the then diocese of Madras.

The journey was a pleasant two week interlude: through the Straits of Gibraltar and into the Mediterranean, a first stop of just a few early morning hours in Port Said and then through the Suez Canal to the heat of the Red Sea. The second stop was Aden, where we went ashore for a few hours and wondered why. It was baking hot and there was so little to see. Then we reached Bombay, early on a Monday morning. After a day spent in an intensely hot Customs shed, we were put on a train for Madras that same evening. We knew – and were told – nothing about how to survive a thirty-six hour train journey and had to wait many months to discover that not every trip by train would be as uncomfortable as that one.

In Madras we were allocated a house called Brightside, whose neighbour bore the name Sunnyside. Were the early missionaries really as jolly (or unimaginative) as their naming of houses suggested? The house had large verandahs, upstairs and down; the ground floor consisted of one large dining/sitting room with a small very basic kitchen off. Upstairs were two bedrooms, beds draped in mosquito nets, with small concrete walled and floored bathrooms off. The big city was all around. The swirl and noise of traffic: buses, cars, auto-rickshaws, swarms of black bicycles and all the while a cacophony of horns.

The first task was to begin learning Tamil and that involved a scooter ride every morning to the cathedral compound where Clara Clarke, wife of the Cathedral Presbyter (and later Bishop) Sundar Clarke, was my first Tamil teacher. Following ordination as a Presbyter on All Saints Day 1964, Tamil lessons were punctuated by preaching in English language churches around the city and pastoral care of the small CSI Anglo-Indian congregation at St Thomas's Mount.

It was not until the end of June 1965, after our first holiday in Kodaikanal and the birth of our daughter Helen, that we moved to Vellore. My first job was to help with Bible Correspondence Courses run by the diocese from an office in the Vellore Mission Compound, and to prepare to take that over from the Revd. Dr Eugene Heideman, who was also Presbyter of St John's Church. In that first year in Vellore we lived in what was known as the Ashram house, in Filterbed Road – a very large house, built around an internal courtyard over which part of the roof could be opened or closed. There was a primary school in the same compound and we soon got used to eating meals with the faces of young children staring solemnly at us through the windows. And we appreciated one of the great advantages of moving to a house previously occupied by Americans; the windows were screened against mosquitos, something that British colleagues of a certain age seemed to regard as an effete practice.

To reach the hospital from the Ashram house on our Vespa scooter, it was necessary to follow three sides of a square. But from the flat roof we could look across directly to the hospital buildings rising above the one and two storied houses and shops between. Anne decided there must be a short cut and set off one evening along a track that seemed to lead in the right direction. She wondered just a little about the people who stared at her from their elevated positions either side of the path – but then people in that part of the town always stared at foreigners anyway. Suddenly she came to a bridge, crossing over the track directly in front of her and at about chin height. Only then did she realize that she had been following the course of a dried up river bed.

At the end of that year, in June 1966, the Heidemans returned to the USA and I found myself taking over both jobs – the Correspondence Courses and Presbyter-in-charge of St John's. In those days St John's had a flourishing and fascinating congregation. About ninety per cent were staff and students of CMCH. There were people from all parts of India from all over the world and from many denominations, as well as CSI, who worshipped together in the English language and in various forms of worship at St John's. It was a most distinguished congregation and a great privilege to minister to such people. There were two services each Sunday, one at 7.30 am attended by students (medical students, nursing students and the whole range of paramedical students who followed courses at CMCH) and one at 9.30 am, to which families came and during which the Sunday School met in the Church Hall. The Church would be full for both services and on the rare occasions (Good Friday and Christmas) when we had only one service, the congregation would overflow onto the steps and the area outside, and listen to the service through the open doors and windows. I recall the competition, in those days before microphones were used, between my voice and those of the crows and monkeys in the Compound. The organization of St John's was also both sensible and stress-free. There was (perhaps still is?) only one committee, the Pastorate Committee, which met once a month and dealt very efficiently with all that needed to be done – except for the worship and preaching, which were left to the Presbyter, aided by the Deacon, Ernest Fritschi and the lay readers. I see from a copy of Sermons from St John's which was signed by the whole Pastorate Committee that the members early in 1971 were:

Paul Christian, Bob Carman, K Barnabas, Peter Hill, I Sigamany, Ramani Pulimood,Mary Poonon, PSS Sunder Rao, Mary Sulakshini, Hannah David, Cyril Jayachandran and K I Koshy

We moved to the Parsonage, a pleasant and sensibly sized one-floor flat, built over the Church Hall and that provided home for the remainder of our time in India. The Fort was not a residential area and in the evenings, once the offices had closed and the courts had risen, it became very quiet (the Temple was then an archaeological site). Behind the Parsonage was the Police Training School and College, where our only resident neighbours lived. Mark was the member of our family best known to the policemen. He was an early riser and from the age of six would get himself dressed at about 6 am and creep out of the flat via the kitchen door (we would hear the screen door slam shut), down the winding concrete stairs to where he kept his bicycle. Then he would go for his early morning ride around the roads inside the Fort. At the same time, the recruits would emerge for drill and PE. One of their routines was to jump over a water obstacle and Mark would watch and wait for the inevitable moment when someone fell in.

When we moved to St John's, Helen was one year old and the Indian luxury of an ayah enabled Anne to return to teaching. She joined the staff of Vidyalayam, the English-medium school for children of Hospital and Medical College staff and taught full-time for the remainder of our stay in Vellore. Our morning routine involved a journey by car (by then we had our gray, Madras-built Standard Herald, about which many stories could be told) to College Hill to drop off Anne and Mark, and I would then drive back along the route as far as Mission Compound to spend the morning in the Correspondence Course office. In due course Helen would be taken to Nursery School (do the children still sing '*The wheels of the bus go rrr-ound and rrr-ound*?'), from where the ayah would collect her at the end of the morning and take her to her own house in Bagayam for a few hours – a wonderful opportunity for cultural exchanges.

In Vidyalayam staff at that time were Betty Baker (the Head Teacher), Ammu Abraham, Mrs Gajapathy, Mrs Barnabas, Mrs Lazarus, Mrs Luther and Anne. When Anne joined the staff there were two classrooms either side of the playground and about sixty children in all. When Helen joined the school there were two reception classes and so a third side of the square was built on to make room for them. The children came from many different language backgrounds and as was the case in India as a whole, it was English that continued to provide the link language. But there were curiosities. The reading scheme was American and it followed that the spelling also had to be American. But an Indian-English lilt and structures borrowed from south Indian language, added to the particular charm of the children's speech. Half an hour a day was set aside for the study of another language and children could choose between Tamil, Hindi or (after Anne's arrival) French. The day began with an assembly and was punctuated by a midday break when ayahs brought tiffin carriers containing lunch, which was eaten sitting on the floor of the Reception classroom.

With Vidyalayam and St John's, our contacts with CMCH staff grew and deepened. Nearly thirty years later we are aware that many of our friends, scattered around the world, are people we

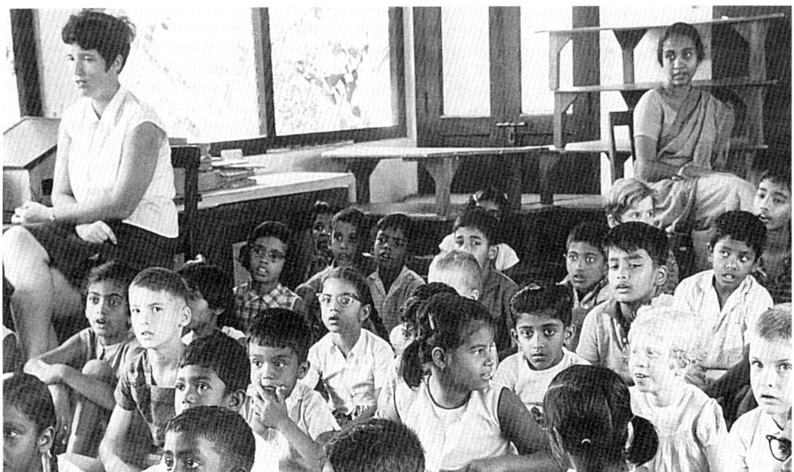

Anne Bishop at CMC School

first met at Vellore. But not only Vellore. The St John's Presbyter was also expected to serve as Chaplain to the Leprosy Hospital and Research Centre at Karigiri. In addition to other visits, I would drive out to Karigiri one Sunday a month to conduct a Communion Service. It was always remarkable to see so many patients – mostly Hindus from villages around – who would come into that beautiful chapel of St Luke at Karigiri, sing the Tamil lyrics, follow the prayers of the Tamil Communion service and no doubt say their own prayers too. The dedication of staff to their work and their patients in that lonely place was remarkable.

St John's represented a highly developed form of ecumenical co-operation. In addition to those who had entered the CSI in 1947, or had been brought up in it since, there was a large number of members of the Mar Thoma Church who had their own Holy Qurbanah once every three months but otherwise entered fully into the life and worship of St John's and made a great contribution to the Church.

Additionally, there were expatriates from all parts of the world who made their spiritual home at St John's but whose home backgrounds represented a wide range of denominations: American Baptists and Lutherans, Canadian Presbyterian's, Anglicans from England and Australia, Congregationalists from Britain and South Africa, Swiss Evangelicals, Church of Scotland, Dutch Reformed … was there ever a congregation like it? I recall that after my first service as Presbyter-in-charge, Paul Stephens, then the organist, said to me: 'It's good to have an Anglican back at St John's'. I took that as a compliment.

Vellore was a remarkable experience, the confluence of three astonishing and amazing things: India, the Church of South India, and the Christian Medical College and Hospital. May they all flourish for the next hundred years!

In the 1970s and early 1980s, Peter Bishop was Chairman of the Friends of Vellore and subsequently has remained on the FOV Executive Committee and as a Trustee of the Vellore Rural Communities Trust. ***CH***

Dr Valerie Major: Anaesthesiology 1967-1995

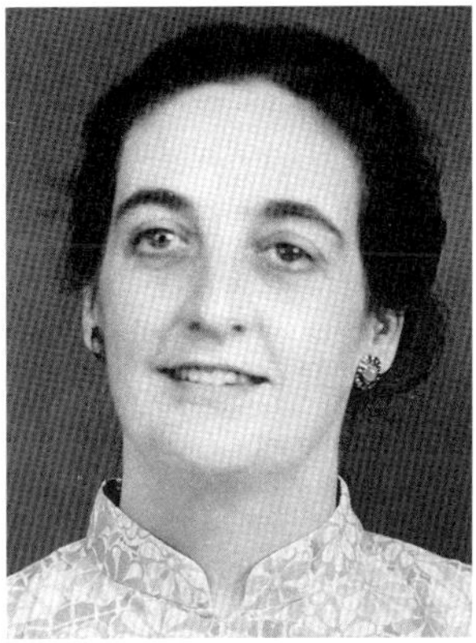

Dr Valerie Major

Dr Valerie Major, who was Professor and Head of the Anaesthesiology Department at CMCH Vellore retired in 1995. She had joined CMCH in 1967 on a Nuffield Research Scholarship and the Anaesthetics Department in 1969, supported by the Church Missionary Society. She was promoted to Professor in 1973 and became Head of Department in 1977.

Dr Major was given the Pask award by the Society of Anaesthetists in Britain for her distinguished Service in India.

She is a Board and Executive member of the Friends of Vellore and her talks to groups of supporters are much appreciated. *CH*

Memories of Vellore by an Occupational Therapist: 1966-1993

by Monica Hopkins

My memories of Vellore began from 1966 when I arrived from England with a large trunk and equally large black box containing a 'cello. I lived at first with the lively family of Webbs and while getting dug into Tamil study was well entertained by Jonathan aged two. This included swimming in a well just beyond the College compound, along with snakes and other wild life – not something I'd expected to do in India. I enjoyed exploring the compound and beyond with the children and this led to my first experience of CMC's medical skills. I had a large thorn removed from my foot by Dr V Benjamin himself at Community Health.

It seemed that my 'cello playing was more appreciated at first than the occupational therapy role I was trying to develop at the Mental Health Centre. The Carmen-Oesterling-Walter clan of musicians were in need of a 'cellist. We began to play together for our own enjoyment and this led to many years of happy music making. However, my cello disliked the climate intensely and revolted on two occasions with a loud bang as a string broke just before we started to perform. This rendered the base line totally absent!

The College choir was another joy and initially challenged my ability to put on a sari for Chapel. I wanted to learn an Indian instrument and at one stage took up the sitar. Mr Navasu, my guru, was a clerk in the Vellore Post Office and unfortunately he was transferred elsewhere before I got very far.

Student and staff entertainments were a great way for the community to get together. I can still see Dr LBM Joseph sitting on the stage cross-legged, wearing only a dhote, earnestly drumming a big mud pot, or "*Dr Malathi*" taking her ward round up the bazaar for her shopping! There were picnics too, ear-bashing bus rides to far distant places, with the odd breakdown thrown in. One to Amoithi Forest remains with me. Diesel was spurting out of the engine somewhat dangerously. But, after a few anxious moments and lots of advice yelled from one end of the bus to the other, this was "*no problem*" as condoms were readily available at a local petti shop. They were purchased and stretched around the offending tube in no time!

Auditory bombardment was a continuous hazard in Vellore but sometimes it hit us more strongly than others. I remember fleeing into my bathroom during long political processions as they passed the College compound and staying shut in for what seemed like hours, to lessen the impact of the noise.

In the early stages of Occupational Therapy's development we were helped by Australian volunteer therapists. They each came for two years and contributed in different ways, both to OT and to the life of the community. Three of them actually met their husbands at CMC. They were full of energy and walking to local hills became a popular activity for us all. A favourite one was to climb Kailas on a moonlit night, avoiding heat and waking up in the morning to see the brilliant sunrise from the top. This was my idea of heaven, except for the times we got lost en route in the dark. Walking of a different kind was Jean Bald's relax-ation, with Suggie her beloved dog, which had been found as a pup by one of the volunteers.

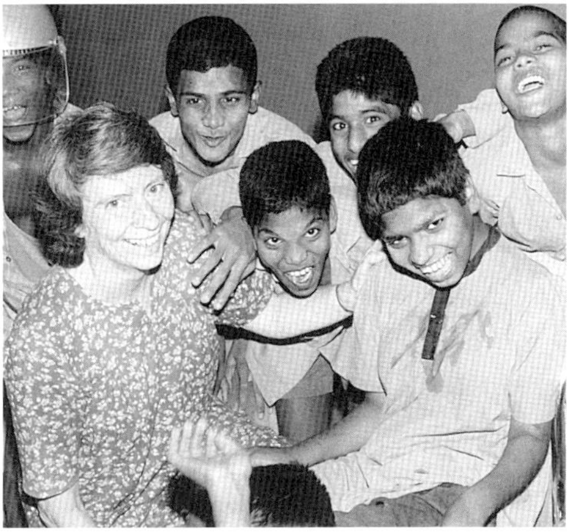

Monica Hopkins at Anbu Illam 1993

My favourite relaxation was to cycle in the countryside around Otterri, Toad Hill and farther afield. I think it was unusual for a visitor to pass through Big Bungalow or the Annex without being invited to join me on one of these trips. It was cooler than walking and we could outstrip any children that tried to follow us.

At Big Bungalow we had the chance to meet so many people over Simon's delicious meals and his entertaining stories. In the late 60s the most notable guest was Granny Brand. She came from time to time in search of her son Paul, when he was over from Carville, USA, for the Karigiri Council meetings. She would totter to the big table with her two bamboo canes supporting her and talk about riding up the Koli hills to "*her*" people who would insist on growing more and more marihuana!

The life of the community at CMC was really something special. We realized this only after leaving it. Whilst there I'm afraid we took it too much for granted. The focus of the community was the Christian faith experienced by many of us and the worship in which we shared. We were able to share a unity that was enriched by the numerous different traditions from which we came and this was a joy as yet still sadly unattainable in our own country.

What of my work? It was full of challenges and this I enjoyed – the fact rather more than the situations! Dr Mary Verghese, who humanly speaking was the reason for my going to Vellore at all, was an inspiration and helping to initiate the Rehabilitation Institute programme in 1966/7 was exciting to say the least. Developing OTs' contributions with Suranjan Bhattacharji and his team more recently was a really satisfying experience which I miss more than anything.

Involvement in the Community Health and Development programme through the OT community rehabilitation team and student Community Orientation Programmes were some of the highlights for me, involving working on creating low cost aids suited to the homes of the disabled people.

Our students were fun, though hard work! As graduates they and the physiotherapy graduates enabled us to become involved in projects beyond CMCH. One of these was the centre for children with cerebral palsy, Anbu Illam, which was taken up by Vellore Diocese of the CSI. An increasing number of children and their families are so grateful for this centre, with which I do keep up some involvement, mainly at a distance.

There is so much to thank God for, especially the continuing development of CMCH and its outreach programmes. And thanks to all at Vellore and for all you have given me.

Some Memories of a Pharmacist

by Rosemary Murchie (nee Sharp) 1967-1983

I first went to work at Vellore in 1967, travelling by sea to Bombay and then on by train to Arkonum Junction where I was met by a welcome party from the Pharmacy with a van to transport my 11 pieces of luggage (including a bicycle in a crate). It was good to meet up with Vic Oesterling with whom I had been in correspondence for some months beforehand and also to see the familiar face of Caroline Moses, previously met in London. I remember being presented with a beautiful jasmine and marigold garland (and being tipped off in a whisper by Caroline not to keep it around my neck as only brides go on wearing them!). After a hot dusty drive to Vellore, John and Alison Webb welcomed me into their home where I occupied their guest room for the first 10 days. I shall never forget my first shower and hair wash in Vellore as, after the overnight journey in the train, I was filthy from all the smuts that had blown in through the open windows (in those days the old steam locomotives were still in use). As the water poured over me, long black rivers of dirt trickled down my body and I felt I really knew what it is like to have one's sins washed away.

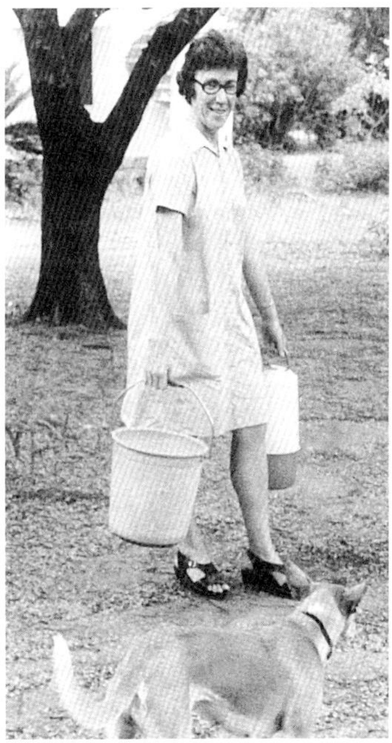

Rosemary Murchie demonstrating the water shortage

That first evening there was a welcome dinner at the home of Ellis and Margaret Carlier (Ellis was an Australian pharmacist) and here I met several more pharmacy staff and began to try to get my tongue around some of the names. Grace and Rachel were no problem. Vasantha was not too difficult, but Navajothimoni almost defeated me and it was a great relief to find she was normally known as Nava. The main problem I had was that everyone looked alike to my unaccustomed eyes and I felt quite ashamed until I found that Indian people going to England for the first time have the same problem.

The first days passed in a blur of heat and whirlwind visits to the hospital to meet staff and see what was in store for me. I had come to set up a quality control laboratory for the pharmacy to provide quality checks on various pharmaceuticals made on the premises, especially the large numbers of intravenous fluids. There were designated premises and even someone appointed to assist me but I was destined to head for Kodaikanal for two months language study and some cooler climate, so work did not start at once.

On return to Vellore we set about unpacking the magnificent set of equipment that Vic had ordered at my request. Finding a home for it all in our 10' x 6' "laboratory" was quite a problem and some had to be kept packed away for a year or so until we got larger premises. The Lab was so small that only one of us could work at a time, but we soon got some simple procedures going and started to set standards for the various products. After about a year alternative accommodation was found for us in Thotapalyam House, a building accessed through the back wall of the hospital grounds and previously turned into a laboratory for the Welcome Research people before they got their own building. We had the ground floor which consisted of three rooms, one of which was actually air conditioned. So all the equipment was unpacked and we really began to make progress. Later the upstairs area was allocated to the Occupational Therapy School.

As is usual in CMCH, one of our roles was to provide orientation and training in our particular expertise for visitors from other institutions. During the time at Thotapalayam House we had some Drugs Inspectors seconded from Mysore State and also pharmacists, both Indian and expatriate. One of the expatriates was a German girl working at Ludhiana who became a very dear friend, with whom I am still in contact. Two of the Mysore Drugs Inspectors were particularly memorable for their enthusiastic approach and we had many interesting discussions during our coffee breaks in the office where the coffee was brewed over a Bunsen burner. One day one of them said, "of course the thing that makes all the difference to this hospital is the temple in the middle" referring to the hospital Chapel. Mr Kusumaker was a Hindu gentleman and we had not been talking about religious matters but his remark really brought home to me how the existence of CMCH and the dedication of the staff speaks to people, really in a far more telling way than anything one can say about God's love and care for his people. I have been eternally grateful to that Drugs Inspector for giving me the phrase "*The temple in the middle*", which has stood me in good stead for many a talk and sermon when on deputation in England.

On the domestic front, for my first six years I had a bedsitter plus bathroom in Big Bungalow Annex at the College Campus and my next door neighbours were Monica Hopkins and Jean Bald, both occupational therapists. The conversation over our meals and during our social time always tended towards "*shop*" and I used to wish I had another pharmacist to talk to at these times. However, I learnt a lot of occupational therapy in the process and thus expanded my horizon considerably. Inevitably my particular work was more of a back room job, working with two or three other pharmacists and I seldom had much to do with patients, so the OTs helped to give me a more balanced view.

One of my enduring memories of my whole time in India is the constant struggle to obtain adequate water supplies. One particular bad year the supply at the college was so poor that there was seldom enough pressure to have it available from all the taps. At one time we had to collect it in buckets from a tap in Big Bungalow and store it in whatever containers we could find. A fund raising campaign was started in England to finance the hospital's pipeline to the Palar River and I was photographed collecting my buckets of water, for publicity purposes. Even today whenever forecasters start talking about drought, a feeling of sick panic starts to creep over me and I have to remind myself very firmly that this will not mean no water in the tap except for two hours in the day but simply that we may not be able to water the garden.

The Quality Control section was not the only part of the Pharmacy to be struggling with inadequate premises and even when I first arrived, plans for a purpose built department were on the drawing board. The area designated was in OPQ Block, which was at the back of the hospital and included operating theatres, dietary and laundry departments as well as several wards. It was exciting to be involved in the planning and to have a say in what facilities would be needed for my own area. On 26th January 1972 we had a grand dedication ceremony with the unveiling of a commemorative plaque. At that time the skeleton of the department was complete but I think only the offices and the in-patient dispensary were actually operational. Quality Control moved in soon afterwards and by the end of 1972 it was all up and running. At that point I departed on extended home leave because of a back problem. Vic Oesterling resigned during my absence and Sujit Das was appointed in his place. John Jayaseelan, one of our graduate pharmacists, took over the quality control work and when I returned in January 1974 I was asked to start a drug information service. This was a completely new departure for me but with the example of Ida Scudder and countless others, who had tackled anything they were asked to do, spurring me on, I struggled to get to grips with a very different aspect of my profession. Before long I became quite absorbed but starting from scratch meant there were no set routines and I was very glad to have, as a secondary responsibility, oversight of the Pharmacy Stores and involvement with the Pharmacy Purchase Committee.

By this time I was living on the hospital campus, sharing a flat with Valerie Major, so I did not have a bus journey to and from twice a day. I enjoyed the feeling of being more at the centre of things but missed the calmer, more peaceful atmosphere of the College grounds. Living with Val, the "shop" talk tended to be more about anaesthetics and since anaesthetics is applied pharmacology I found this a really useful back-up in my work with Drug Information. As a result of the move to the hospital, being a more senior member of staff, I was given a master key and asked to provide emergency back-up during the night when our night duty staff ran out of some essential item or met with a problem they could not deal with. Fortunately, I did not get called out very often but I have memories of hurrying through the hospital grounds, keeping a sharp eye out for the enormous bandycoots that tended to prowl about at night and murmuring a prayer that I would be able to cope with whatever had arisen.

The back problem persisted but eventually, largely due to Valerie Major anaesthetizing a patient of Dr Jacob Abraham's with similar symptoms and making the connection, a proper diagnosis was made. Surgery was scheduled for January 1975 but a few days before that the 10 week strike at the hospital commenced. This was a quite horrendous experience which I hope we never have to go through again but at the same time I feel glad that I went through it and survived it. We learnt a lot in the process and there were lighter moments. I shall never forget Sr Marlienne Tomson's face as she was helping us out in the dispensary when I brewed up coffee on a Bunsen burner using a pyrex beaker borrowed from the lab and sweetened it with Syrup BP, all stirred together with one of my glass stirring rods.

A few weeks after the strike ended, plans for a visit to Australia to study drug information services there came to fruition and I took my first journey south of the Equator. For my stay I was hosted mainly by people who had worked in Vellore: John and Sally Rothwell, Ellis and Margaret Carlier, Reg and Beth Walker, who all set out to give me a really good time as well as making sure that I got the information and experiences I needed. The Vellore network spreads wide and everywhere you find such welcoming and co-operative people, it is really heart warming. When I returned to India, as well as the knowledge gained, I took enough money in donations to start equipping our library with the right books, filing cabinets, etc, and plenty of contacts to whom I could turn when I needed further help.

Shortly after I returned my back surgery was re-scheduled and in August I became an in-patient and saw the hospital from a very different perspective. Everyone was very kind and helpful and I made an uneventful recovery. Since then I have had over 20 relatively pain free years and I am eternally grateful to CMCH, Dr Jacob Abraham and Valerie Major for solving a problem that defeated even Harley Street.

Further changes in senior staff in the Pharmacy saw the departure of Sujit Das to the USA for study leave, from which sadly, he never returned. His place was taken by Dr K L Hemnani who had spent 10 years in the USA and was a very different person from previous Chief Pharmacists we had experienced. However, he was very keen to see the department continue to progress and I was soon able to adjust my modus operandi to fit in with his ways. One of our problems over the years has been finding and keeping suitably qualified and experienced staff capable of running the department. People were sponsored for higher studies but most of them once they had worked out their bond (and sometimes even earlier) left for better posts elsewhere, usually in the Gulf countries. The reason for this was generally family pressures and the need to provide for children, or brothers and sisters, rather than a simply personal desire for more money. In the extended family set-up prevailing in Indian society this is very understandable but it did not help us to build up a good senior administrative body in the Pharmacy Department. The expatriate staff in general saw themselves as people who passed on such expertise as they had to Indian colleagues and then moved on. Several times I thought I had reached this point only to have the person concerned move on instead of me. However, by 1982 it appeared that Dr Hemnani was going to be a permanent staff member and circumstances at home in England suggested that maybe the time for me to move on had arrived. On 11th April 1983, 16 years to the day after I had arrived in Vellore, I left and returned to England. For me working at Vellore was one of the most formative experiences of my life. The opportunity to be involved in the work of the institution was a great privilege and the chance to meet and work with such highly motivated people was an unforgettable experience. The NHS seemed very tame by comparison.

Reading through what I have written I am struck by how much more there is to say. I have not mentioned so many people who played such an important part in my experiences: Joel Davanesan who was the first pharmacist appointed to assist me but who sadly died from the effects of chronic diabetes. John Rothwell, a young Australian pharmacist, who brought a breath of fresh air with his easy natural friendliness to all and sundry (and who was influential in my learning to play Bridge, for which I always will be grateful). My dear friend Chandra whom I first knew as a student, who has been sponsored twice for further training and now occupies a very senior position in the department. She keeps me in touch with current trends and we have been able to help from time to time with input from here. It was lovely to have her staying with us at weekends while she did three months work experience in England – a small return for the wonderful hospitality I received in India.

I could go on writing for months but I hope these few reminiscences will be a useful contribution to the collection being made to mark the centenary.

Thirty Years As Part of the CMCH Family

by Ann Bothamley – Nursing Sister

How can one ever express in a few lines the events, experiences, challenges, heartaches, joys and opportunities of being part of the CMCH family for 30 years?

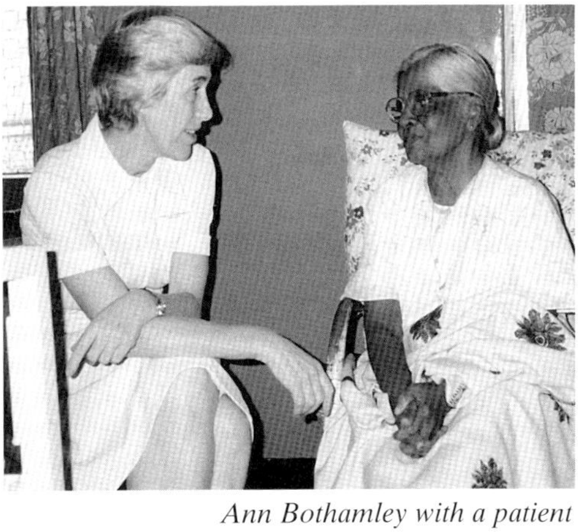

Ann Bothamley with a patient

Seconded by the Baptist Missionary Society in 1968 to work in the capacity of a nursing sister brought many challenges and opportunities from planning and staffing and setting up new units (Coronary Care, Renal Transplant and Bone Marrow Transplant) and redesigning parts of 'M' Ward, to running the laundry with Marliene Thomson and twelve medical students at the time of the strike. There were Hospital Administration students to teach, Bible classes for interns and student nurses, protocols to write and Chapel prayers to take.

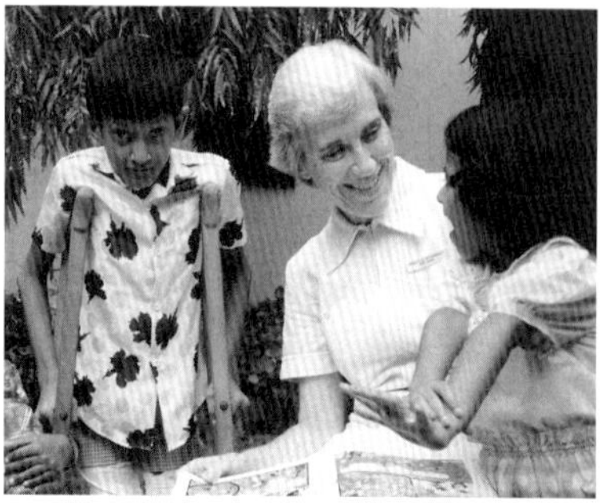

Ann with young patients

Opportunities abounded and were there to grasp, from fostering medical students, making birthday cakes for my much loved Leukaemia children – for sharing the joys and sorrows of the staff in the 'M' Ward family – for raising money for poor patients each Christmas and sitting with those who were dying.

It wasn't always easy – the numbers of relatives I would cajole into the lift, only to find them smiling at me as again they made their way up the stairs!, or the monkeys who seemed too quick and clever for any of us. The medical staff always seemed to need a bed when there wasn't one but were sure I could do something and the relatives and patients who were convinced I could solve any problem from a leaking tap to their speedy discharge

My life in Vellore was enriched by teaching a girls' Bible class at St Johns for 24 years, fostering medical students, being involved in musical activities and work in the Sweepers' and Rag Pickers' villages.

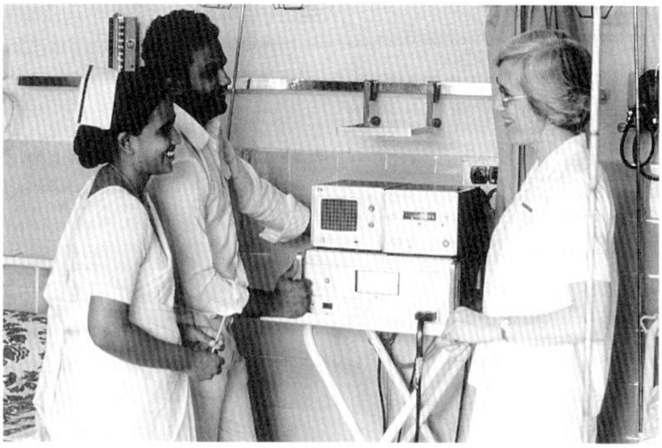

Ann Bothamley on the ward

In 1981 I was faced with the problems of CMC doctors working in the rural areas of India and concerned about the education of their children. The

Balanilayam Trust was formed and Marliene Thomson and I took the first children into our flat in Anandagiri. In January 1990 we opened a purpose built home for these children who are educated at the Ida Scudder School, thus enabling their parents to continue Ida Scudder's vision for the people of India.

A kaleidoscope of colour, of events and experiences of people I came to know, respect and love. It has been a great privilege and an opportunity to share God's love with those who indeed became my brothers and sisters.

Occupational Therapist At CMCH 1968-1983

by Jean Bald

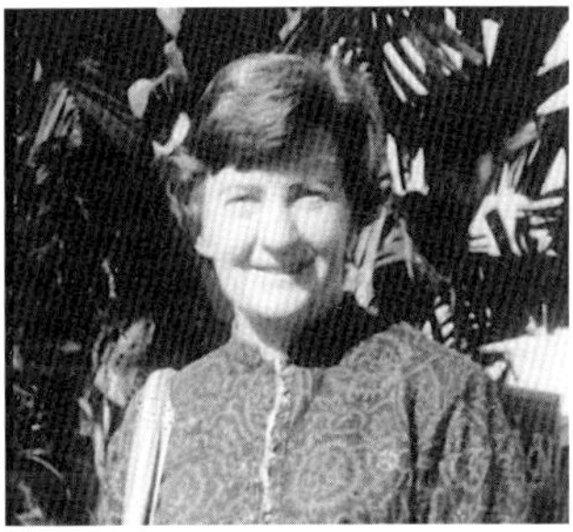

Jean Bald, c. 1980

To cover 15 years in Vellore in a few words is not easy but I'll try to highlight my most meaningful experiences.

My arrival was auspicious to say the least as the heavens opened over Arkonam Station and Monica Hopkins (who was meeting me) and I were drenched. Dried out on the bus ride to Vellore, we had a second drenching as we reached the Medical College and I was introduced to the Principal and his wife, Susie. My colleague Monica helped me with induction to life at Vellore, where we planned and initiated the course of Occupational Therapy.

At first we battled to get students to register – Occupational Therapy was an unknown quantity! The confidence of the College and in particular Dr K G Koshy as Principal, paid off in the course of time and before I left we had recognition by Madras University of a 3 year degree course with 6 months' internship thereafter; we had four clinical areas of Occupational Therapy and could select students from many applicants. In the first few years we were greatly helped by a succession of Australian volunteer occupational therapists who manned the clinical departments and taught students.

In 1995 I was happy to return for the Silver Jubilee of this course, to find that all the staff were Indian – products of CMC – and new buildings had arisen for education and treatments in the hospital. I remembered the classrooms at Thottapalayam House into which 6 students and a teacher just fitted! I remembered digging our own clay for pottery classes, scraping the leaves of the katali (sisal) plant to make fibre (and incidentally to exercise upper limbs of stroke patients). I remembered the garden with a thatched hut where our patients practised domestic skills in village style, our little garden beside the great Wellcome Building, the Community Health camps when our students joined with the medical and physiotherapy students for village practice. I remembered too the opportunities to participate in research and work with Dr Mary Verghese, Dr Jacob Abraham and Dr Selvapandian. It was wonderful to be part of the developing Mental Health Centres and the teamwork, which included patients and their family members along with the staff.

I realize how blessed I was to have spent those fifteen years in Vellore. Never before or since have I been privileged to live and work along with so many dedicated people. The College bus to St John's Church of South India at the Fort on a Sunday morning full of medical students for the 7.30a.m. service, or children and parents for the second service, represented the joy of belonging to that huge Christian family.

The 1970s

AN ANAESTHETIST AT VELLORE 1969-1979

by Dr Ruth Mansfield MBE

After retiring in 1967, I thought I would like to continue my profession as a cardiothoracic anaesthetist overseas, using my experience at the Brompton and other chest hospitals. In 1969 I went to Vellore in south India, initially for one year but I continued there intermittently until 1979; and from 1980 to May 1981 worked at Wanless Hospital and Miraj Medical Centre. Both of these are mission hospitals.

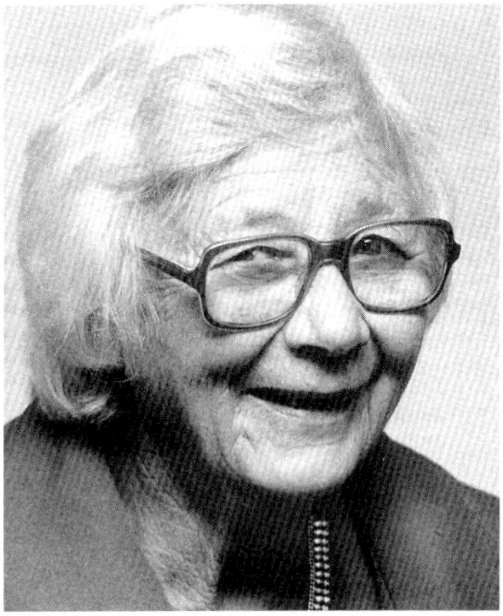

Dr Ruth Mansfield

My interest in India was first stimulated by an aunt, Dr Florence Payne, who worked before and during the first world war in Ludhiana. Later, a friend, Dr Gwenda Lewis, organized the anaesthesia department at the Christian Medical College, Vellore, where she had contracted poliomyelitis but carried on from her wheelchair until 1966, when I visited her. It is encouraging that medical women in India are well represented at their own India Medical Women's Association, as shown by an attendance of 400 at a meeting in Madras of the State Branch.

When I arrived at Vellore there were six operating theatres, of which two were air conditioned but after a new engineering department was built in 1973 to supply medical gases, compressed air and air conditioning, a theatre complex of fourteen theatres, seven anaesthetic rooms, recovery area and sterilising rooms was built, each unit using two theatres at a time. This put a strain on the anaesthetic department with only four senior staff and trainees for the MD and DA. By the efforts of Dr Valerie Major from Cardiff, the trained staff increased to eight with the MD in Anaesthesia.

Operating started at 7.30am, which meant being there at 7am, if it was an open-heart case, to check drips and drugs that had to be prepared before bringing the patient into the theatre, particularly if it was a child. There were often shortages especially of disposable needles, i.v. canuli, sometimes drugs and medical gases and cost had to be considered. The air conditioning often broke down, particularly in the summer. I was mainly involved with anaesthesia for the cardiothoracic unit and particularly with their open-heart programme.

Dr Ruth Mansfield MBE

by Clare Howes

Ruth Mansfield, MBE, anaesthetist, died at her home near Haslemere on December 10th 1994 aged 92. She was born Ruth Webster in London on August 1st 1902.

Ruth Mansfield was Consultant Anaesthetist to the Brompton Hospital for Diseases of the Chest from 1948 to 1967. She was widely respected in the medical profession for her expertise in giving local anaesthetics for the operation of thoracoplasty for pulmonary tuberculosis. Known to all her colleagues as "Mrs M", she undertook sessions at sanatoria in Surrey and King Edward VII Hospital, Midhurst, with visits to Sully Hospital near Cardiff.

She co-edited a textbook on thoracic surgical anaesthesia and was the author of several papers on the subject. She took part in the early work on open-heart surgery as a colleague of Lord Brock, Sir Clement Price-Thomas and many other well-known surgeons in that field.

Ruth Mansfield was married in 1925, the year before she qualified in medicine and spent the next seven years working for the

Red Cross and as clinical assistant at the Belgrave Hospital. While bringing up her family of two, she became house anaesthetist at the Westminster Hospital; inspired by the late Sir Ivan Magill, she decided to make her career in anaesthesia.

After working in the Emergency Medical Service during the Second World War at the Mayday Hospital, Croydon, and the Chest Unit at Horton Hospital near Epsom, she was appointed assistant anaesthetist at the Brompton Hospital and became a consultant there in 1948 at the beginning of the National Health Service.

Her wish to help others in less fortunate circumstances led her to work voluntarily in Hospitals in Malaysia and Israel and after her retirement from practice in this country in 1967, she spent ten years at the Christian Medical College Hospital in Vellore in southern India, with only short visits home. While at Vellore she introduced anaesthesia for cardiac surgery and for this work she received the MBE in 1977. At the age of 77 she spent two years at the Miraj Medical Centre, Maharashtra.

She and her husband were Nonconformists: neither of them drank or smoked but they never forced their views on others and were most generous and kindly hosts to their younger colleagues and their families. Ruth Mansfield enjoyed playing tennis, gardening and swimming, the last two well into her eighties.

She never lost her interest in anaesthesia and on the day of her death, attended a meeting on the history of anaesthesia at the Royal Society of Medicine and delighted her colleagues with spontaneous recollection of her experience in dental anaesthesia over fifty years ago.

The Friends of Vellore were privileged to have Dr Ruth Mansfield as a member of their Executive Committee and Board. She attended our last Annual Reunion in September 1994.

CH

Vellore Concerts

by David Chesterman

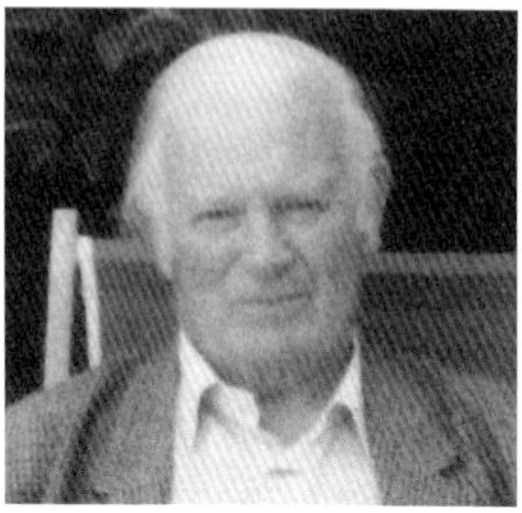
David Chesterman

I took over the management of the Vellore Albert Hall Concerts when that redoubtable and lovable man, Albert Jefcoate, retired from this task after many successful occasions.

One of our most regular early soloists was the pianist Eileen Joyce, who was renowned for playing three Concertos in an evening and changing her dress between each – green for Mozart, yellow for Grieg and red for Beethoven.

I had been a Vellore supporter for many years and my father, Sir Clement Chesterman, had been Chairman of FOV. The Albert Hall Concerts had started in 1951, and the London Philharmonic Orchestra was always hired but the time came when the cost of employing a professional Orchestra became excessive. I suggested that the only way to produce a reasonable surplus on the Concert was to use a good amateur Orchestra which would give its services or make only a modest charge. I was then working for the Ernest Read Music Association, and will never forget their Orchestra's first appearance for FOV at the Albert Hall under Terence Lovett, in one of the largest choral works in the repertoire – the Berlioz Te Deum, with a huge battery of percussion and a choir of 600 voices from the Home Counties. At the end, where most composers set the words "*Let me never be confounded*" very quietly, Berlioz does the reverse. With blazing brass and the organ flat out, he tells the Almighty that he, Berlioz, will never be confounded! At this Concert, because we had such vast forces available, we included the Vaughan Williams setting of "*All people that on earth do dwell*" so we really had a choir of 4,000.

Other memorable occasions featured "*The Dream of Gerontius*", Delius's "*Sea Drift*", Walton's "*Belshazzar's Feast*" and Beethoven's Ninth Symphony, in which he urges all men to be brothers. There was an occasion when John Lill, giving his services, like all other Vellore soloists, played Beethoven's Choral Fantasia and the Fourth and Fifth piano Concertos, after which we had a party. About midnight John remarked: "*David, I feel a little tired, I think I'll be off*". Hardly surprising, having played, with rehearsal, the equivalent of six concertos in a day!

Sadly, as the years went by it became more and more difficult to fill adequately a hall the size of the Albert, with many more competing concerts going on, so it was agreed to adjourn via the Festival Hall, to the Barbican. Our last Concert there included, appropriately, Mendelsson's "*Hymn of Praise*", ending with the words "*All things that have breath, praise the Lord*".

Apart from thousands of pounds, which accrued to Vellore from these Concerts, they did give FOV a chance to acquaint a larger public with the invaluable work it was doing in India, as well as providing a highly enjoyable social occasion.

We owe a great debt of gratitude to all the conductors, soloists, singers and players who made these Concerts possible, and I am glad that the tradition still continues in the classical Concerts which still take place annually in Birmingham.

The Revd Joseph Pratt: St John's 1974-1992

by Valerie Major

The Revd Joseph J Pratt, who died in October 1999, served as pastor of St John's Church, Vellore for nearly 16 years. He went there in November 1974, having been ordained in the Rayalseema Diocese of South India and serving in Jambalamadugu for 6 years and then Anantapur for 7 years. He returned to the UK in 1992 and along with Suguna, his wife, continued his ministry in the United Reformed Church until 1998. During his time at St John's he also shouldered the chaplaincy at CMC hospital during three periods of leadership vacuum there.

Joe Pratt was a great believer in careful planning and organization, with meticulous attention to detail. He realized that for a church like St John's, with a considerable floating membership, it was important to establish traditions and so developed these at Advent and Christmas, Lent and Easter, All Souls Day and Harvest Festival. The St John's Prayer Book was one of the lasting contributions to the infrastructure of the church. He also loved the building, so when the woodwork began to collapse, he encouraged the congregation to consider a total rebuilding. The new light and airy church is another memorial to his time there.

Joe believed, and said, that if you gave someone responsibility they would grow into it. He made certain that a large number of the congregation were actively involved in church life, acting as ushers, hosts, PCC members, convenors and committee members, taking prayers and reading. St John's probably has the largest number of lay readers of any CSI church, and half of these are women. He started the area fellowships where more informal friendships could develop. He also started a link between St John's and the United Reformed Church in Lancaster which meant that on several occasions people from Vellore visited there and the minister and members of the congregation from Lancaster visited Vellore

Above all Joe was a pastor, available to all who turned to him – and his gentleness and friendliness meant that many did. There are many of us from the congregation who will always be grateful for his quiet and prayerful support, as will the Friends of Vellore, whose Annual Reunion services he conducted in the UK.

THE US AMBASSADOR AT BIG BUNGALOW

by Peter and Christine Hill (CMCH 1970-1980)

For the last two of the ten years that we spent in Vellore, we lived in Big Bungalow on the College Campus. It was a lovely 2-storey stone house, built around a central "well" that was open to the sky and had originally been Dr Ida Scudder's home. As well as now being home for us and our three children, it was the College Guest House with six rooms for visitors. Christine was responsible for the Guest House which involved managing the comings and goings of many guests as well as overseeing numerous College dinners and other functions that were held in the large open plan lounge and dining area on the ground floor.

The Chief Guest at Graduation in 1979 was the American Ambassador to India and, of course, he was booked to stay in Big Bungalow with his wife. The Consul from Madras and his wife were also guests of the College for the night. Their security man came too – he shared a room with Jonathan our youngest son, as all the guest rooms were full!

Soon after our guests had retired to bed – early after a busy day around the Hospital and College – we heard a truck stop on the main road, followed shortly by the sound of marching. Imagine our surprise to find ten or twelve armed reserve police with rifles and bayonets at the front door of Big Bungalow. They had come to protect our important guests through the night.

With help from the Ambassador's security man, we persuaded them to make their HQ for the night round the back of the house, rather than on the front porch. The official party were all trying to sleep in the rooms above the front door and we felt that the clunk of heavy boots, belts and rifles all night would not be conducive to peaceful sleep, however much it might enhance security. Obligingly the policemen settled down on the back verandah, leaving their rifles inside the front door for safekeeping. One of them kept guard at the front but exchanged his boots for a quieter pair of rubber chappals.

Our guests left in the morning, having assured us that they had enjoyed a restful night – but to our horror, after they had gone we discovered a dead bat on the floor in the room which had been used by the Consul and his wife!

Peter and Christine Hill worked in Vellore from September 1970 to June 1980 with their children Jeremy, Katie and Jonathan. Peter was Professor of Clinical Biochemistry.

The 1980s

Lord Coggan and Lord Runcie

In the year 2000, the Friends of Vellore have lost two distinguished Vice Presidents who had been leaders of the Anglican Church: Lord Coggan and Lord Runcie, both had close links with CMCH Vellore.

The Most Revd Lord Coggan of Canterbury: Lord Coggan will be particularly remembered for the teaching missions he lead at CMCH Vellore in 1980 and 1989. The sermons he preached there were published as "*The God Who Heals*".

The Most Revd Lord Runcie of Cuddesdon: Lord Runcie's visits to CMCH Vellore in 1986 while he was Archbiship of Canterbury was a brief but memorable one, as outlined in the Friends of Vellore Newsletter of Spring 1986.

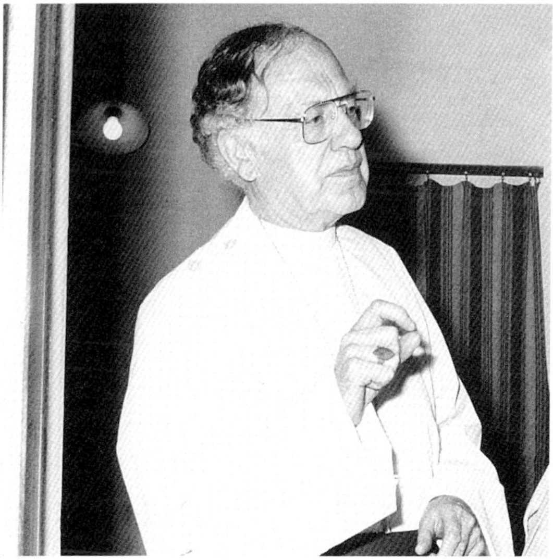

Lord Runcie at CMCH

Vellore Service: Radiation Physicist 1981-1983

by Christopher Green

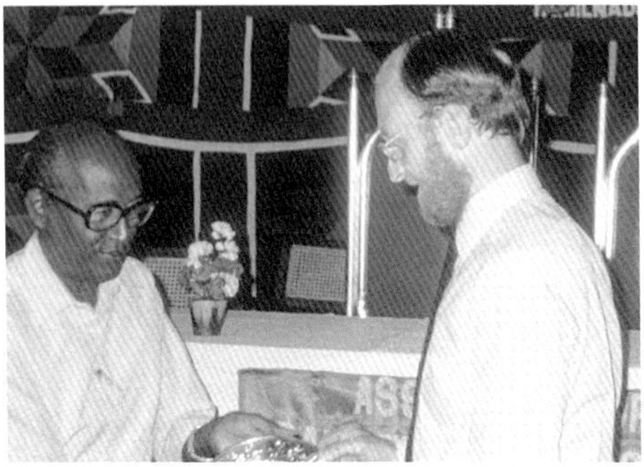

Dr Christopher Green at conference of Radiation Oncologists of India

There came a point in my life when I wanted to do a period of service in the Third World; I offered myself to VSO and was accepted for Sierra Leone but my Church's assistant Minister, Barbara Stanford, suggested the Baptist Missionary Service. I was very warmly welcomed and they immediately thought of CMCH Vellore, where they already had a missionary, Ann Bothamley, who was the senior nursing sister in charge of 'M' Ward. The BMS thought I was suitable to go straight out; it was only a case of waiting for a visa to go out as a missionary. In the end, I waited 18 months for a visa which was then refused, the first time Vellore had had a visa refused. Instead I went out as a Volunteer with no salary, for which I didn't need a visa and approximately two years after I first applied, I was about to fly out to India to go to Vellore. I reflected that I could have gone out to Sierra Leone with VSO and completed two years service in the time it took me to get to this point.

I was to join Dr Cyril Jayachandran, Professor of Radiation Physics in the Isotope Laboratory, part of the Radiotherapy Department, helping and advising in Nuclear Medicine. Fortunately, Ann Bothamley was returning to Vellore at the same time with another BMS missionary and I was to fly out with her from Heathrow on 8th December 1981. Over-night, how-ever, there was a huge downfall of snow and I was two hours late getting to Heathrow, the plane was delayed for five hours and the pilot arrived after me! I met up with Ann in the Departure Lounge and we flew out stopping at Dubai and arrived in Delhi to find that my luggage was still in London: on to

Madras, met by Marliene Thompson, a 100-mile drive to Vellore. I was taken to Brian and Ann Witchalls' where I slept and slept!

Everyone was very kind but it didn't stop me suffering from culture shock and terrible homesickness, which I'd never had before in my life (I was 35 at the time). Very soon, my accommodation was ready and I joined Jean Bald, Heather Payne and Monica Hopkins in the Big Bungalow annexe, where an Australian Nuclear Medicine Technologist, Valerie Reid, was to join us soon after. She already worked in my department, and made important contributions to its running.

Cyril Jayachandran invited me over for a dinner party very shortly after I arrived and I went with my colleague, Mr J V R Rose, his wife Selva and daughter Dolly. Walking out in the still night air afterwards with Dolly, I was astonished to see that the crescent moon was flat on its back and exclaimed "*The Moon's the wrong way up!*" and Dolly replied "*What's wrong with it? It's always like that*". I then realized that a few degrees change in latitude would result in an equal number of degrees rotation of its phase.

It was close to Christmas and I was invited to 'Cottage Prayers', which was a cross between a social and a prayer meeting at people's houses, taken in turn, monthly. I think we sang carols and I can recall '*Joy to the World*' most vividly, because I had never sung it before and I loved it. Poonoose Matthews was the host and I met the Carmans for the first time there. Some of the Priests thought that westerners were automatically endowed with gifts of preaching or extemporary prayer and could sometimes call on you without warning: drop you in it would be a better phrase! Once, at Cottage Prayers a Priest opened proceedings with, "*I call on Dr Christopher Green to lead us in prayer*" and I managed to stop my jaw hitting the ground, say a few solemn prayers slowly, hoping the long pauses would somehow sound holy and thoughtful, before privately running out of ideas and launching into the Lord's Prayer. An American missionary friend and his wife once went to a local Tamil Church to see what it was like but found the two hour service heavy going and were actually sneaking out when they were stopped by one of the local worshippers with "*Where are you going? Brother has just sent word that he wants you to give the*

Message!" And so they had to. Twice I was asked to take the hospital early morning services for the nurses for a week at a time, and did so, though they usually arrived in dribs and drabs: I'm not sure that they were wholly gripped by my addresses.

Most of the Christian staff, Indian and expatiate, attended St John's Church in the Fort, where I enjoyed my first service and was muted on by a crow as soon as I left! That wasn't repeated, fortunately and I enjoyed the services at St John's for the rest of my time in India. In the evenings, the College community would go to the service in the octagonal College Chapel, where I would usually try to sit in the same seat on the right, from where I had a good view of the mountain Kailash through one of the windows. The service always started in daylight and it was quite black outside at the end of it. The service always ended in the same way: the lights would be suddenly snapped off and in the dark outside, with only the everlasting candle light shining in the Chapel, the choir would sing the blessing "*The Lord bless you and keep you …*" and so on to the end. I always found this electrifying.

I soon fell victim to bacillary dysentery, and was admitted to 'M' Ward feeling dreadfully ill and wretched but was fortunately under Ann's care. I was visited by Dr A Singh and the entire Radiotherapy team, which was rather nice and also by Jean and Ian Todd (later President of the Royal College of Surgeons). They were neighbours for a short while on the College campus and I had actually staggered to their house that morning before I was admitted. They knew I didn't particularly like dogs, rabid or otherwise, as in India the dogs often fight at night and the noise is dreadful. One night the noise was so bad I turned over in bed and thought that one of the wretched dogs was surely being disembowelled. Jean Todd later told me that at that moment, she had turned over to Ian and opined that I must have been out there disembowelling it personally. I didn't think I would survive a month in India but somehow I did and got used to everything and made many friends.

My principal job was helping Cyril in the Isotope Laboratory with its general work and sharing in lecturing in radiation physics to postgraduate radiotherapy doctors studying for radiotherapy qualifications and I particularly enjoyed that. The lab work was more in the nature of slow, steady progress but things gradually got done, getting air conditioners and the Betatron Bed fitted with emergency power lines, for example. The power supply started to exercise me and dominate my thoughts, as many will know. The Hospital would usually get at least one power failure a day without warning, sometimes more and if the power to advanced electronic equipment failed on load, it would damage it and the computer had several boards blow out. I advised fitting a motor-starter switch to the computer and this was done immediately and although it didn't stop a power failure, it did stop power surges damaging the computer when the power came back on again. With the encouragement of the Medical Superintendent and Valerie Major, I was invited by the Deputy General Superintendent to do a survey of the hospital to ascertain the power needs of each department and this I did with Chitteranjan Reddy and George Vergese, with the object of finding out who needed an uninterruptible power System (a UPA) Class 1 power, who needed just an emergency power line (Class 2), and who could make do with ordinary mains (Class 3). The survey was completed and I made my recommendations, but failed utterly to convince the Directors that it was necessary.

Although the cost of a reliable American System was probably less that a tenth of the money spent on the CAT scanner, the idea failed to fire their imagination and expensive equipment continued to be bought or given to Vellore and continued to be wrecked by its power system. I continued to harp on my hobbyhorse and no doubt got myself a bad name during this period. I helped in problem solving in lots of little ways. Once I went into the 'Eldorado' Cobalt Unit with Mr Rose to find everyone wondering what to do about the treatment area light source which has just failed and which meant that they couldn't use the machine. It turned out that one of the light bulb's power supply lines, which was physically rather like a steel tape of the kind found in tape measures, had become disconnected and had coiled itself up tightly, right down a tube into the machine. I can recall saying immediately "*you need something like a wire coat hanger*", and wondered where I would find one, turning round to find one hanging on the wall behind me. With everyone looking on, fascinated, I undid the coat hanger and bent it into a long wire still with the hook at one end and fished down into the tube and hooked out the coiled steel tape. I lost it again but on the second attempt secured it carefully and got the electrician, Mr Anamaly, to take over and fix it permanently. Everyone seemed very impressed!

One thing I was asked to do was to teach Fortran Programming, and this I did. The Hospital had recently acquired a computer from America, really for accountancy purposes but tax wasn't payable if it was to be used for research, so the hospital authorities were anxious to encourage the staff to use it for this and hence asked me to teach a few classes. Many departments asked me to do this and at one point, I was commuting back and forth on public transport between hospital and college giving one lecture after another to different departments. I taught Philip Korula in particular and after I left and returned in 1989, I realized that he had long since overtaken me in computing expertise. I was shocked, of course, to learn of his untimely death sometime later. Towards the end of my time in Vellore, Keith Hall, a real computer scientist, came and took over my classes and really got things moving.

I managed to see a bit of India, visiting all four major cities, Bombay, Calcutta, Delhi and Madras and right at the end of my two year stint, did a northern tour and going to Varanasi, Delhi and Agra, seeing all the sights and really enjoying myself. In Delhi Ann Bothamley suggested that I stayed at the Community of St Stephen, which she thought was an order of monks who permitted guests to stay. Actually, it turned out to be an order of nuns but they were quite happy to have me anyway and I have stayed with them since. I managed to combine the northern tour with acceptance of an invitation from the British High Commission in Delhi to a Garden Party on Tuesday 22nd November 1983, where I was presented to the Queen and the Duke of Edinburgh; a great honour. I don't think I particularly deserved it: I had attended a few meetings at the Deputy High Commission in Madras and so was just a name known to them when they were asked to suggest expatriate names to the High Commission in Delhi.

I can recall that I wanted to be back in Vellore for my birthday, (27th November), and made it back in time. Shortly after I went to my last Cottage Prayers and at the end I was talking to Molly Thomas, who asked me what the two years had been like and how I felt. I felt a little depressed and thought I hadn't achieved very much but Molly was quite encouraging and said that I'd made a lot of people aware of things and indeed, when I later returned in 1989, I was delighted to find that many of my suggestions had been followed.

I had a gentleman's agreement with the Baptist Missionary Society that I would serve two years and so in late December, arrangements were made to fly me back to Britain on a 747 (I had asked for this experience) and had an uneventful 12 hour flight to Heathrow where I was met by David and Nora Shapton, friends from my church, who put me up for a week. I can recall being surprised when the Captain of the 747 announced that we were now 'over the Baltic' at some point in the flight but realised that a Great Circle route would be the shortest, and would track over the Baltic from Delhi to London.

During my time in Vellore I had doubts and often wondered about whether I was really called to serve there but when I returned to England I felt a much stronger sense of believing that it was where I was meant to have been.

All that was over 16 years ago but I have never forgotten my time in India, and have been to nearly all the FOV Annual Reunions since. I have kept up a number of friendships, especially with Mr Rose and family and was delighted to be invited back in 1989 for the 50th Anniversary special Conference of the Radiotherapy Department at Vellore. I had none of the earlier homesickness, delighted only in being there but I still got ill again! I can't do much to support CMCH, but I am asked occasionally to meet someone at the airport, or help with finding the odd bit of equipment, so I'm pleased to help in these smaller ways whenever I'm able to. Was it all worth it? Yes: I may have achieved very little in the end but I gained a great deal and learnt a great deal and I feel the bonds between our nations are worth more than any material gains. There really is a warmth in the family of Christ that we all share in CMCH and in the FOV, more precious, as they say, than any jewels.

The 1990s

Young British Volunteers From the 1990s at CMCH

by Dominic Jenkin

As a Schools' Partnership Worldwide Volunteer, I was one of the two chosen from my school and I was pleased to know that I had a worthwhile activity to occupy the major part of my future year off before university. In retrospect, I believe my attitude towards the trip was wrong; I was excited, of course, but with selfish intentions. That may seem a strange thing to say when I thought all I wanted to do was help, yet how could I help when I didn't even know what I was going to do? How did I expect to cure a problem before even knowing the symptoms: only in arrogance. Maybe if I had gone as a teacher I could have educated some children but only in part; as a nurse I could have stopped a cut from going septic but only those presented to me. After I left, it would not be my place to help but someone else's.

I was assigned to help in the Rehabilitation Department at the Christian Medical College and Hospital at Vellore and on arriving was officially made Recreational Therapist, along with my partner, David Keown. Patients at the Institute commonly suffered from spinal damage, resulting in partial or total paralysis of limbs, or other neurological or cerebral disorders, also resulting in total or partial paralysis. Ironically the place I had been sent to contained only the incurable. Quadraplegia and paraplegia is something I had never thought about before I went to India, doubtless because of its futile nature. Never to be able to play those favourite games again, never to be able to run, to swim, to dance, never to be able to toilet oneself again, or to be independent. Suddenly words like never, can't and help became common usage. "*I'll never*", "*I can't*", "*please help me*".

One of the patients, a year younger than myself, was a keen cricketer. He had a great ambition, which, it seems might have been fulfiled. He wanted to play for India, until he awoke one day and couldn't move his right leg. How can he but feel despair? Another patient, Lalan, told me, "*but life was so good to me before*".

As my stay passed, so too did my naivety. What I realized was that I was not the teacher, the doctor, the helper, but I was the pupil, the patient and the needy one. I learnt that all I was able to offer was love, that most valued above all commodities. But I also found out that it was a long time before I could stop learning.

I spent three and a half months working at Rehab, extended from a stay originally planned to last three months. No, for once the apparent delay had nothing to do with Indian bureaucracy but was a representation of David's and my own feelings: we liked the place so much we didn't want to leave.

India has contributed greatly towards my present attitudes, for which I am grateful. It is a country no different from ours, or any other. Like every country it has one great redeeming feature, that of love. When I left, there remained behind many friends and memories of good times. To me it is not the place which is important; man can build nothing to compete with nature's splendour but certainly it was the friends I made along the way who were the real enjoyment of India and many were at CMCH, Vellore.

David Keown

Dominic and I have both very much enjoyed working in the CMC's PMR Department (Physical Medicine Rehabilitation). The Rehab Institute involves physio and occupational therapy and we spent most of our time helping out in the latter. We were free to work in either but it was quite evident to us that we could be most helpful to the three Occupational Therapy Staff. This is because they have a lower staff/patient ratio and our strength was useful to them when it was necessary to transfer patients from their wheelchairs on to their stretchers. OT also involves simple bits of apparatus used to exercise or strengthen the limbs or muscles for a practical use, i.e. increasing grip of the fingers so that the patients will be able to eat unaided. The workshop that adjoins OT has a complete set of carpentry tools where apparatus can be constructed or duplicated when necessary. This requires a greater degree of determination and initiative than knowledge of carpentry.

Our role in the Occupational Therapy Department developed with time and experience. Not being qualified, we have not been able to be OTs. Nevertheless, we learnt a number of techniques for supporting and shifting patients which means that the OTs have more time to concentrate on the actual treatment and on those patients that are more demanding. In fact, we have become known as the 'Recreational Therapists' – when we had the time we were very happy to entertain the patients with a variety of games. There are great opportunities for physical games – the department possesses javelins, shot puts, footballs, badminton, a table tennis table, darts, a carrom board (the Indian equivalent of snooker) and after one of Dominic's earlier projects in the workshop, a complete set of skittles. Otherwise there are all sorts of passive games – chess, draughts, Connect-4, playing cards, solitaire, numerous jigsaws and children's games and my workshop achievement, a jumbo sized Kensington board, with various coins rather than little counters. This enables patients who have limited grip, to play the game. There are many resources which can be used in a number of original ways. However, new games brought from England were always gratefully accepted (Connect-4 was a recent introduction and has become very popular). The work here need not include any work in the workshop as there is always plenty to do.

Suranjan Bhattacharjee, Head of PMR believes that in a department where the emphasis is on treatment, another important element of healing can be neglected – making sure patients are happy and encouraging them to realise that despite severe disability, life can still be enjoyed. So one of my main aims was to help this aspect of healing and to prevent patients feeling useless, or uncared for. Luckily, despite the increasing reliance on technology in hospitals around the world, care is still universally recognized as an essential constituent in the healing process by everyone involved with medicine.

I'm now back in Vellore, spending my final two weeks working in Rehabilitation again. It's great to be back, there are still patients here who were here when I left in May and it is good to be reunited with all the friends I have made in the CMC. Just a final note of further thanks: I very much appreciate the fact that you made this possible for me. I have not only found the "experience" that I was seeking but more importantly, I have had a wonderful time. No doubt I will be returning to Vellore in the near future.

Speech Therapist 1994

Amanda Howett

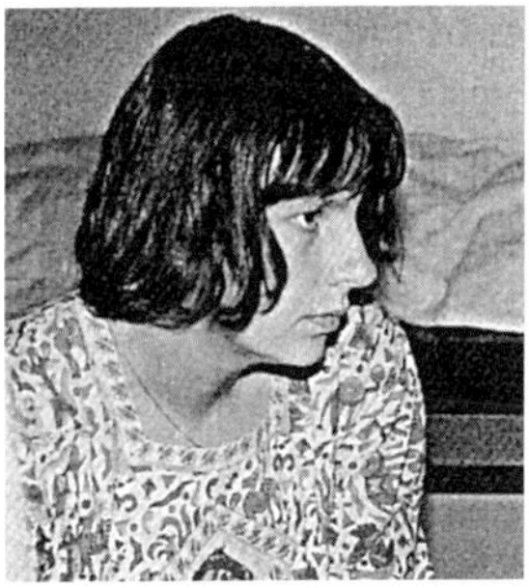

Amanda Howett

I went to CMCH on a Church Mission Society Experience Placement, a scheme for young Christians to experience and work in a different culture. So I flew out not really knowing what the place would be like, who I would meet or what I would do.

So how does a monolingual English speaking Speech and Language Therapist benefit from and try to contribute to the life of a large Indian hospital? Good question. Well obviously language is quite a problem. Apparently there are 14 major languages in India and with CMCH attracting patients from all over the country, most of these languages are represented. Even by the end of my time, my Tamil and Hindi were not beyond the level of questions such as "*what is that?*" and names for body parts and a few every day objects. So in terms of assessing patients and carrying out therapy I was very reliant on other people to translate for me. People seemed very willing to do this and for me, a very independent person, this taught me a lot. At first I found it very hard taking Speech Therapists, Physios, O.T.s and teachers away from their own work but eventually I felt that getting people involved was the best way to pass on information, as well as providing an opportunity for us to work as a team and for friendships to develop.

I worked with children with learning difficulties at Nambakkai Nilayam, children with Cerebral Palsy at Anbu Illam and with adults in the Rehab department and in ENT. I also did some basic level teaching. Speech Therapy at CMCH tends to be very variable. Sometimes there will be five Speech Therapists in post and other times there will be none. The opportunity of greater financial rewards in government hospitals or overseas often draws people away from CMCH. It would be great to see stability in the Speech Therapy Department and one vision for the future is to run a course to train Speech Therapists. Having teachers and students would then provide a committed core of staff to create such a stable department.

Although I was only at CMCH for nine months, the whole experience has made a profound impact on me. Working in a Christian community where all our work and all our patients were daily committed into God's hands was a real privilege. I realise what a special institution it is. Living in a country where people matter and worth is about who we are and not what we own or what we do, had challenged the values I hold in my British society. I am certainly aware that I gained far more than I could ever give in those nine months.

So I now have my memories of a wonderful time at CMCH and dear friends who I keep in touch with. There are challenges which I hope continue to shape my life now. But one special aspect of CMCH is that it's an international community. I love meeting up with other people who are going to Vellore or who have been there and it's always wonderful to meet up with Indians from CMCH who are visiting or living in the UK. I just hope my hospitality can begin to match that which I was so freely given in Vellore.

I went back to CMCH for a couple of weeks at Easter 2000. I had a great time and it was wonderful to be back in the community, even for a short time. It was lovely to catch up with so many friends. I was partly working, setting up a link between CMCH and the University of Central England where I am now working. Three of our Speech Therapy students are going to CMCH for six weeks at the end of June. It is a great opportunity, which I'm very excited about and so are the students.

MEMORIES OF AN ARCHIVIST

Oliver Wooller – CMCH 1995

There is a special magic about India. The land is sometimes so lush and verdant. The towns are so full of noise and bustle. Everything seems preternaturally alive. Even the CMC Hospital has its own special brand of vim not to mention vigour. In this atmosphere the most mundane events lend themselves to colourful descriptions. The grim work of cleaning, fumigating, sorting, weeding and listing the dust-covered and insect infected records of the Directorate may have been dull beyond boring but I can honestly claim to have seen the dirt in the files on practically everyone in both college and Hospital; touched it; been covered in it and washed it off afterwards. Of course, my lips are sealed but I will say that some people have been applying for leave rather frequently over the years! As for those documents that are preserved, I hope that when future researchers come to read through them in our cool, clean, aseptic, well ordered Archives Library, they will appreciate the efforts that went into making it so.

Then again, why should they? It will not be the work that I will remember but the people, their friendliness, hospitality and infectious enthusiasm. This is true not only of the senior staff who have shown me every consideration and much kindness but also of the students and even, or even especially, of the ordinary people whose knowledge of English is often as restricted as mine is of Tamil.

The Archives project itself – establishing an Archives Library, cataloguing and properly storing the records of the College and Hospital – has made real if unspectacular progress. The two most important departments have had their files listed. I am confident that Dr Alice Kuruvilla (in charge, Archives) and my able trainee Mr C Irudayaraj will be able to continue the work. The only real disappointment is the lack of much really first class early material (pre 1947) amongst the records but then one never knows when some might turn up and we would be pleased to hear from anyone who knows where records from 1901-1947 might be stored. I return to England with many happy memories of Vellore, which I will be more than happy to share.

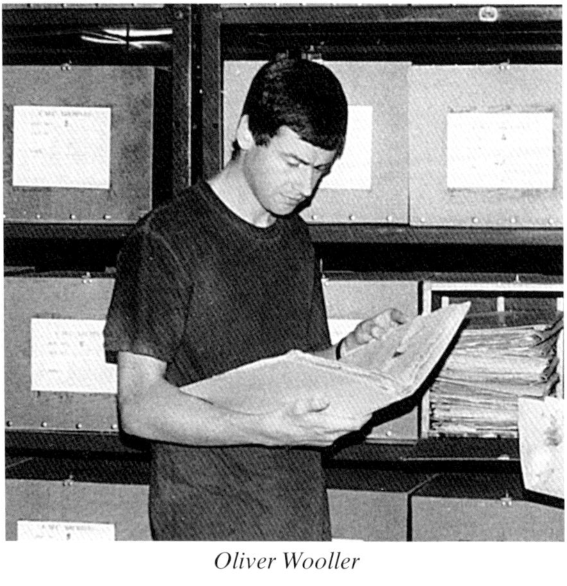

Oliver Wooller

BRITISH PERSONNEL IN THE 21ST CENTURY

The Flemings

Joe and Denny Fleming have now been at CMC in Vellore for over a year. The hospital would like them to be involved for the next five years. Joe is undertaking consultancy in the department of Clinical Biochemistry and Denny has set up home and helped out in the department of Clinical Pharmacology.

They have been married for fifteen years and met while they were both working in a Clinical Pharmacology laboratory in a hospital in Leicester. Joe has been working for the past few years in St Bartholomew's and the Royal London Hospital. He has been in the NHS for over 20 years, has a PhD and is a member of the Royal College of Pathologists. He and Denny have previously worked abroad for two years as lecturers in a medical school and hospital in Ghana, West Africa. However, India and CMC are very different from their previous experience!

As well as giving lectures, Joe has been asked to implement policies for departmental safety and help Clinical Biochemistry comply with the standards being set for the registration of clinical laboratories within India. He is also surveying the services currently offered by the department.

Prior to coming to India, Denny worked for four years in the pharmaceutical industry, then for a charity as a universities and colleges student worker. On arrival at CMC, she has found her expertise very much in

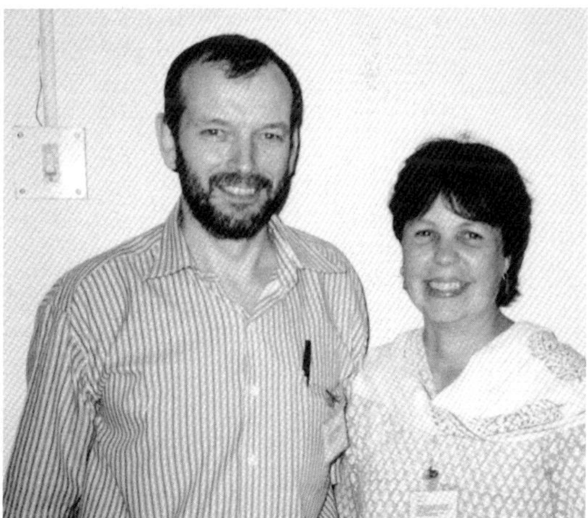

Joe and Denny Fleming

demand. As well as lecturing she is currently helping the department of Clinical Pharmacology assess and expand their low cost manual tests for measuring the blood concentrations of therapeutic drugs.

They are both developing relationships with staff and students and are hoping to have an open home for the campus students. Their presence in Vellore has been arranged through Interserve England and Wales and is partly funded by the British Friends of Vellore.

Other British staff now working at CMCH, Vellore are:-

Richard Chilman, a researcher and facilitator in the Rehabilitation department who has spoken at FOV meetings,

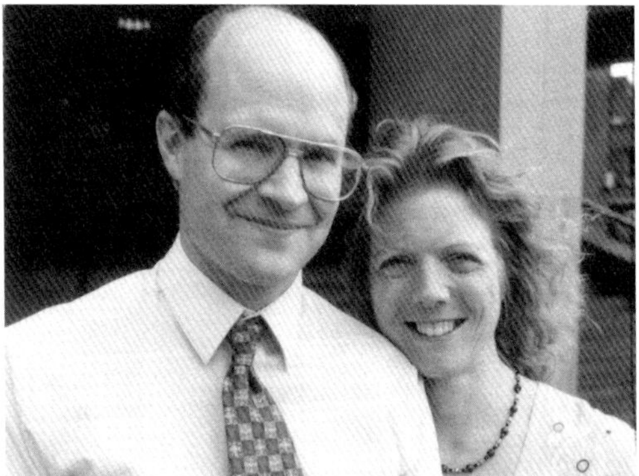

Hugh & Debbie Skiel working at the Account Department and PMR, and Judith & Tony Sykes working at the School and the Engineering Department.

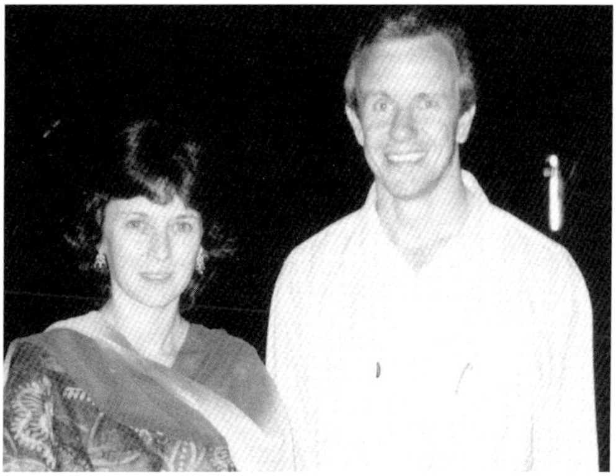

They, together with the Friends of Vellore in Britain and Ireland, will continue the Links of Love which bind us to CMCH, Vellore, into the new Millennium.